In Touch With Your Breasts

The Answers to Women's Questions About Breastcare

In Touch With Your Breasts

James Davidson, M.D. · Jan Winebrenner

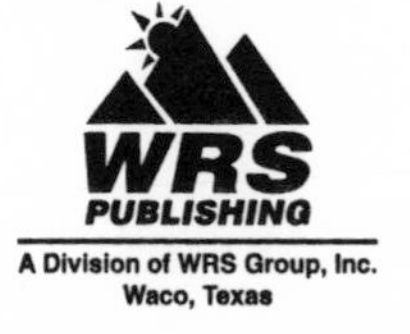

A Division of WRS Group, Inc.
Waco, Texas

DEDICATION

To my wife, Carolyn,
whose humor and joyful giving
define love for me every day.

First published in the United States of America in 1995 by WRS Publishing,
A division of WRS Group, Inc., 701 N. New Road, Waco, Texas 76710
Book design by Stephen Ott and Colleen Robishaw
Jacket design by Joe James
Illustrations by Kent Boughton, M.S.M.I.

10 9 8 7 6 5 4 3 2

Library of Congress Cataloging-in-Publication Data

Davidson, James A.
In touch with your breasts / James Davidson, Jan Winebrenner.
p. cm.
ISBN 1-56796-048-0
1. Breast--Diseases--Popular works. 2. Breast--Cancer--Popular works. 3. Breast--Diseases--Miscellanea. 4. Breast--Cancer--Miscellanea. I. Winebrenner, Jan. II. Title.
RG491.D38 1995
618.1'9--dc20 94-30838
CIP

ACKNOWLEDGMENTS

JERRY LEE BARKER, M.D.
Medical Director, Radiation Oncology
Presbyterian Hospital of Dallas
Clinical Instructor, Southwestern Medical School, 1978-1994
Assistant Professor Radiotherapy, M.D. Anderson Hospital, 1976-1978

JEANICE JANES, R.N.B.A.
Nurse Coordinator
Women's Diagnostic and Breast Center
Presbyterian Hospital of Dallas

PAM JENKINS, M.S.
Rehabilitation Counselor, Department of Psychiatry
Presbyterian Hospital of Dallas

PAMELA J. JENSEN, M.D.
Staff Pathologist, Presbyterian Hospital of Dallas
Clinical Instructor in Pathology, University of Texas
Southwestern Medical School, Dallas

BRYAN H. PRUITT, M.D.
Plastic Surgeon
Presbyterian Hospital of Dallas

BRADFORD F. REEVES, M.D.
Radiologist
Medical Director
Women's Diagnostic and Breast Center
Presbyterian Hospital of Dallas

MARGARET SUNDERLAND, M.D.
Medical Oncology & Hematology
Presbyterian Hospital of Dallas

TABLE OF CONTENTS

FOREWORD

> *"...The clamoring for information is straining existing sources and spawning new ones. Calls to the National Cancer Institute's 17-year-old cancer hotline have surged to 600,000 calls a year from 120,000 in 1980; more than a third are about breast cancer..."*
>
> —The Wall Street Journal
> *May 9, 1994*

When cancer was found in my own breast, of course I was frightened. I cried and experienced all of the reactions you would expect of a woman diagnosed with a life-threatening disease. But I had an advantage that my sister Suzy, whose life was finally ended in 1980 by breast cancer, didn't have—an advantage that we now all have: more information about the options and where to go for answers.

Today's women, who are more informed than any other generation, want to take an active role in the care and treatment of their disease. To do this, mothers, sisters, daughters, and wives are intent upon learning, from whatever sources are available to them, how not to wait passively for a miracle. How not to hope so much as to act in their own behalf. This year alone, nearly 160,000 women will be diagnosed with breast cancer. More than 45,000 women will die from it. In addition to cancer, countless women will face multiple other breast diseases, and their concerns increase as medical professionals continue to stress self-examination, doctors' examinations, and mammography. The subject of breast health is of vital interest to women of all ages and is an ongoing concern ever present in most women's minds throughout their lives.

Dr. Jim Davidson, one of Dallas/Fort Worth's most respected surgeons, knows this, and his practice thrives because he not only treats his patients with utmost professional skill, he is devoted to their encouragement (giving of courage) and their education regarding all matters of breast health. And now he provides women everywhere with basic information—a beginning point and knowledge upon which they may formulate a plan of action.

This book is a contribution of the highest order to preventive medicine. To Dr. Davidson, and to the men and women who are cherished members of our cause, who have helped, each in his or her own way to make life better for all women and their families, a warm thank-you.

—Nancy Brinker
Founder and Chairman, Susan G. Komen Foundation
Author, *The Race Is Run—One Step at a Time*

INTRODUCTION

Every day scores of patients come into my office, bringing a vast assortment of concerns and conditions to be explored. But they all bring one thing that is the same: They all bring questions. Questions about their health. Questions that, when answered clearly, will enable them to make informed and responsible decisions about their health.

Of the many patients I see every day (more than 1,400 new patients every year), at least one-half are women who have been sent to a surgeon for consultation about breast health. They may be concerned about a mass that was revealed on a mammogram, or maybe they discovered a lump during breast self-exam, or they may be suffering from any one of a variety of breast conditions that need the attention of a physician and/or surgeon. In every case, the women I see have serious concerns that trigger questions. Many questions.

This book was written in an attempt to answer many of those questions about breast health that women have brought into my office and into the offices of other physicians who have contributed to the different chapters. The answers given are "middle of the road" answers and, as is true in any field of study, not everyone will agree with all of them. However, most physicians will be in agreement with much of the information presented here.

Certainly, this book is not meant to be a substitute for seeing a physican, but it can act as a catalyst for other questions as you think through matters of your own health, and perhaps it will guide you in communicating with your own personal physicians, as you ask them to elaborate on some of the answers found here.

—James A. Davidson, M.D., F.A.C.S.

Chapter One

ANATOMY AND PHYSIOLOGY

Q. How soon after conception do breasts start to develop on a baby?

A. Breast development begins as early as the 5th week of life, when special skin begins to change into breast tissue in an area called the milk line.

Q. **My sister's baby had milk coming from his breasts after he was born. Is milk from a baby's breasts normal?**

A. Milk can be expressed from the nipples of most babies of either sex at birth. This milk is called colostrum (slang is "witch's milk") and is the result of high levels of the mother's hormones stimulating the baby's undeveloped breast tissue. The milk and mild swelling of the breasts will usually disappear in several weeks.

Q. **At what age do a young girl's breasts start growing?**

A. The age that breasts start developing varies from culture to culture. In our Western Culture, breast development starts about two to three years before a girl starts to menstruate, or at about age 10. At this time the nipple begins to become pigmented and elevated.

Q. **What determines breast size?**

A. The size is determined by the amount of the three types of tissue that make up the breast: the number of fat cells, connective tissue cells, and breast ductal and glandular cells. Genetics and the woman's age determine how much of each type of tissue a woman has in her breasts. For a woman in her twenties, about one-third of the breast is composed of fat tissue; connective tissue comprises about 50 percent or more; and 10 percent to 35 percent of the remaining tissue is composed of breast ductal and glandular cells. After a woman passes her mid-thirties, the amount of glandular tissue in her breasts starts to slowly disappear and the connective tissue and fat tissue increase. After menopause, the proportion of fat tissue to connective tissue increases. By the time a woman is in her seventies, only 5 percent of her breast is composed of breast ductal cells or glandular cells.

Q. **Do any exercises increase the size of the breasts?**

A. No. Some of the apparatus that are sold with the promise to increase breast size actually increase the size of the pectoralis muscle. Because this muscle lies under the breast, its enlargement may make the breasts appear slightly larger.

Q. **I have a mole on my chest that looks like a nipple. Could this be an extra breast?**

A. Extra nipples (polythelia), especially occurring under the breast, probably occur in 1 percent to 2 percent of all women. They seldom cause any problems.

Q. **During my pregnancy I developed lumps under my armpits which became tender. Are these lumps breast tissue?**

A. Yes, they can be. The armpits are a common location for extra breast tissue that does not have nipples. During pregnancy, this tissue can become quite large and painful; however, it is not particularly prone to becoming cancerous. It should be removed only if it is painful. The occurrence of breast tissue in the armpits is seen more frequently in India than in other regions of the world.

Q. **My left breast is larger than my right breast. Is this normal?**

A. Minor differences in breast sizes are found in 60 percent of women. The left breast is usually larger than the right. Anisomastia is the term applied when there is a large discrepancy in size.

Q. **A neighbor's 18-year-old daughter has breasts so large that she can hardly stand up straight. Why are her breasts so large?**

A. Excessive growth of the breast tissue in teenage girls is called juvenile or virginal macromastia. Exactly why it occurs is not known. A surgical procedure called reduction mastopexy can be done to reduce the size of the breasts.

Q. **My 76-year-old aunt has breasts so large she has difficulty finding a bra. Her breasts were not this large when she was younger. What can be done about this problem?**

A. Macromastia, or the gradual enlargement of breasts during adulthood, occurs because of a slow increase in fatty tissue. As a woman ages, the breasts' duct and glandular cells die off and are replaced by fat cells. Treatment for macromastia begins with weight loss. If this does not bring satisfaction, breast size can be reduced by reduction mastopexy.

Q. **When I was younger, my breasts did not sag. Why have they become "droopy?"**

A. Sagging breasts (ptosis) are the result of changes associated with both aging and pregnancy. During pregnancy, the skin and supporting connective tissue become stretched. In the normal process of aging, the supporting connective tissue of the breast is reduced. Suspensory ligaments between the lobes of the breasts, called Cooper's ligaments, lose support as the breasts' firm collagen fibers are replaced with more elastic fibers. The aging process also causes the breast to lose large volumes of breast duct and glandular cells. Unless fat tissue replaces these cells, breasts will become flaccid or flat.

Q. **Is it normal for a woman to have hair on her nipples?**

A. Hair is normal on the periphery of some women's nipples.

Q. **What are the bumps on the skin of my nipples?**

A. The little raised areas of the nipple's skin are Montgomery's glands or sebaceous glands. Both are specialized glands which lubricate the nipple. ***(See diagram of breast, p. 5,6.)***

Q. **How is the breast structured so that milk can be secreted?**

A. The inner structure of the breast is best compared to a tree, or several trees. The trunks of these trees, as many as 8 to 12, empty into the nipple. The breast's ducts are like tree branches, and the glandular cells (acini cells) that make the milk are like leaves.

The breast is composed of 20 to 25 lobes or segments. Each lobe is composed of multiple lobules which are groups of grape-like clusters of cells called alveoli, or acini. The acini secrete milk into ducts where myoepithelial cells contract to propel the milk along the path toward the nipple. ***(See diagram of the breast, p. 5,6)***

Q. **When my nipples are stimulated, one nipple protrudes and the other one inverts. Is this normal? It has been happening for years.**

A. The nipples have muscle cells in the skin that contract with stimulation. Usually both nipples will respond the same way. If one nipple has changed and begun to respond differently, it could be an early sign of cancer. However, if the nipple has always inverted with stimulation, there is no need for alarm.

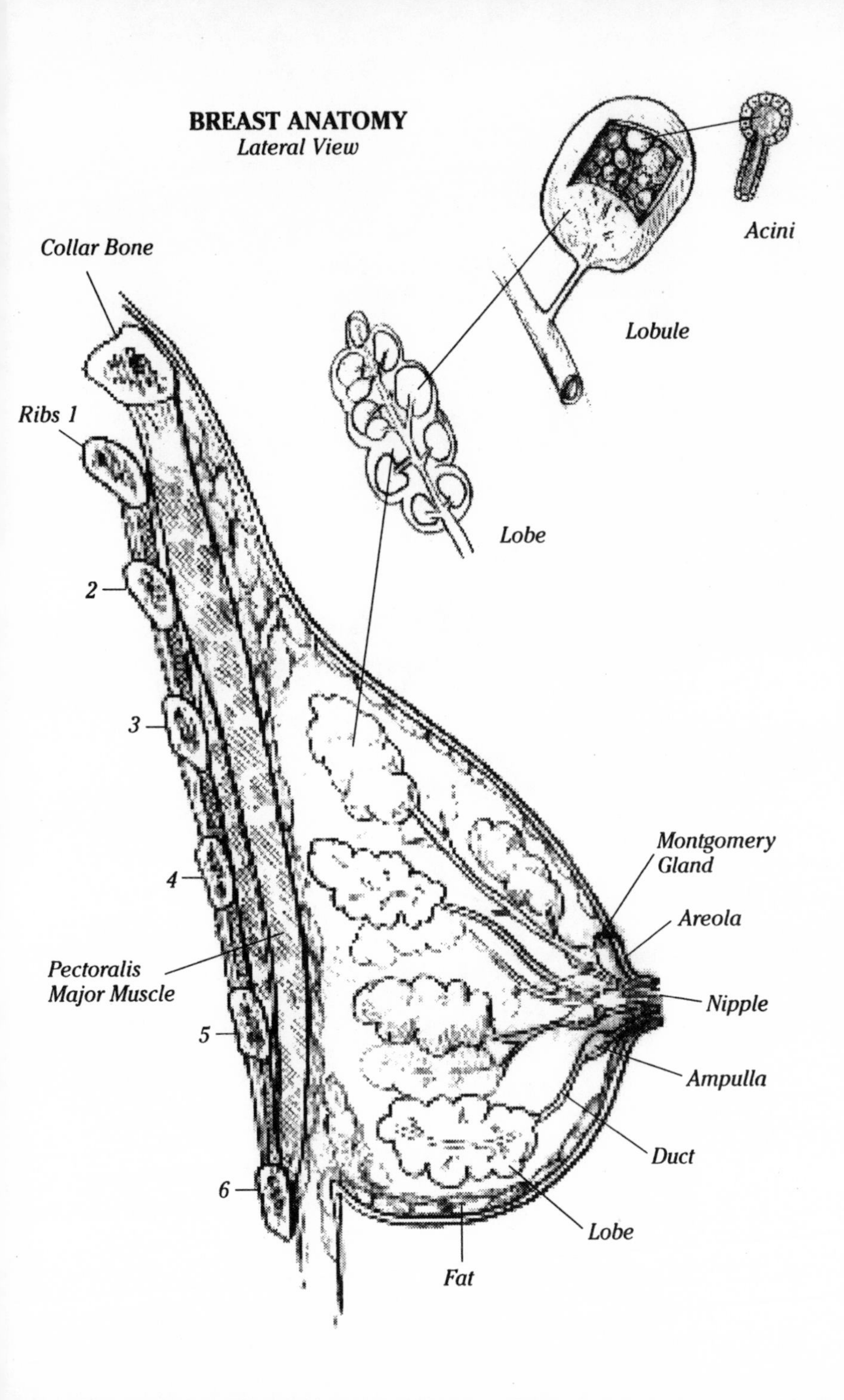
BREAST ANATOMY
Lateral View
Acini
Collar Bone
Lobule
Ribs 1
Lobe
2
3
Montgomery
Gland
4
Areola
Pectoralis
Major Muscle
Nipple
5
Ampulla
Duct
6
Lobe
Fat

BREAST ANATOMY
Front View

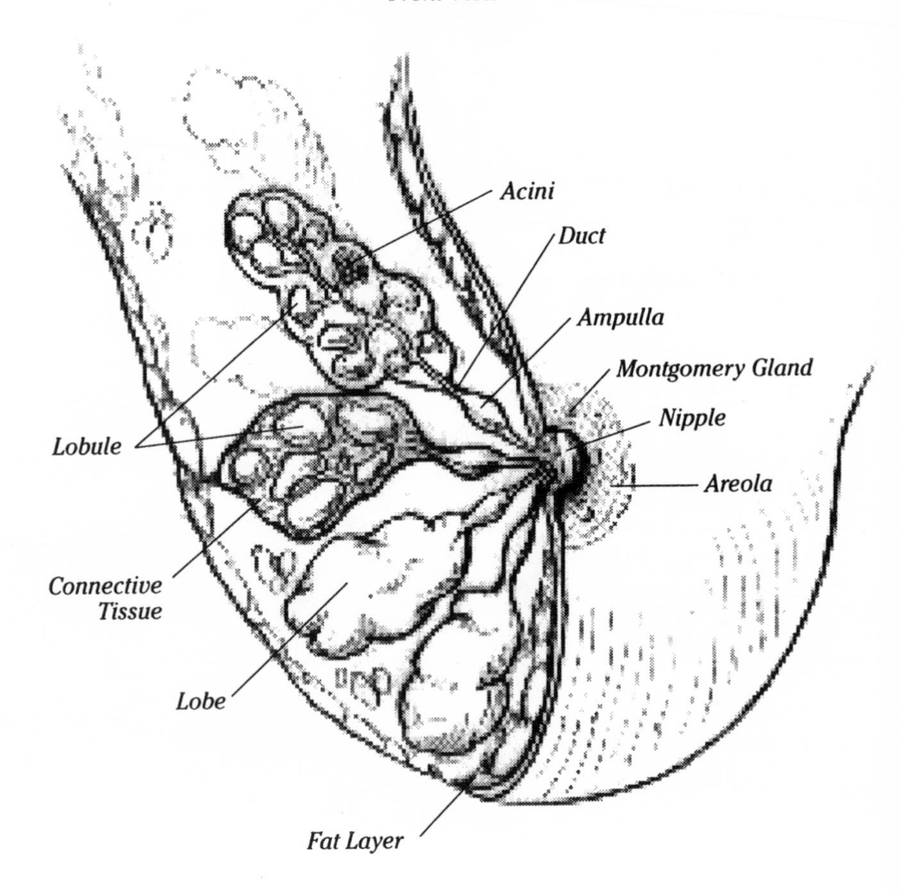

Q. **My nipples have always been inverted. Should I be concerned about this?**

A. Inverted nipples occur normally in some women. These women sometimes experience problems breast-feeding and have more infections of the nipple.

Q. **My 14-year-old son has enlarged breasts. Is this normal?**

A. Approximately two-thirds of teenage boys will have some breast enlargement during puberty (gynecomastia). It is believed to be the result of disproportionate amounts of estrogen and testosterone. This condition is normally resolved, however, before a young man reaches age 20.

Q. **My grandfather has enlarged breasts. Is this normal?**

A. As a male becomes older, an imbalance between estrogen and decreasing male hormone (androgen) levels can occur. This imbalance can lead to breast enlargement. Breast enlargement can also be caused by tumors which secrete estrogens, kidney and liver disorders, and some drugs. A man's risk of breast cancer does not increase if he has enlarged breasts; however, if the enlargement is not symmetrical, that is, if only one breast is enlarged, male breast cancer does become a concern.

Chapter Two

CANCER RISK AND PREVENTION

Q. How many new cases of breast cancer occur in the United States each year?

A. Approximately 180,000 cases of breast cancer in women are reported each year. In addition, approximately 1,000 cases of breast cancer occur among men each year.

Q. **Is the rate of incidence of breast cancer the same worldwide?**

A. No. It's higher in Western countries. Studies indicate that as a country becomes more Westernized, the rate of breast cancer incidence increases. Asian countries have the lowest rate of breast cancer; however, when an Asian woman moves to the United States, her daughter's risk increases and the incidence of breast cancer begins to approximate that of white U.S. women. Many authorities feel this increase in Western countries may be due to a diet of increased fat or possible increased caloric consumption in childhood. Worldwide, the incidence of breast cancer is increasing at a rate of approximately 2 percent per year.

Q. **I have read in magazines and newspapers that my chance of developing breast cancer is about one in ten or one in eight. Is my risk really that high?**

A. That figure is misleading. The chance of the average American woman developing breast cancer in her lifetime is approximately one in eight to ten if she lives to 100 years of age. Since very few women live that long, there is not necessarily a 10 percent to 12 percent chance a woman will develop breast cancer. Every woman's risk is less or greater than the one in eight to ten quoted by the media because each individual has her own personal risk factors—and the figures quoted by the media generally encompass the entire population.

In 1993, *Science* magazine reported the following data regarding the risk of developing breast cancer, by age:

By Age (years)	Risk
25	*1 in 19,608*
30	*1 in 2,525*
35	*1 in 622*
40	*1 in 217*
45	*1 in 93*
50	*1 in 50*
55	*1 in 33*
60	*1 in 24*
65	*1 in 17*
70	*1 in 14*
75	*1 in 11*
80	*1 in 10*
85	*1 in 9*
ever	*1 in 8*

Q. **Is race a factor in the development of breast cancer?**

A. To some extent. Black American women have a slightly higher incidence of breast cancer, up to age 40. However, from age 40 to age 75 and upward, a white American woman's incidence of breast cancer increases while a black woman's decreases.

Q. **How many people die of breast cancer each year in the United States?**

A. In 1993, 46,000 women and 300 men died of breast cancer in this country. Approximately one woman dies of breast cancer every thirteen minutes. It is the most frequent cause of death for women 35 to 55 years of age.

Q. **How can I prevent breast cancer occurring in me?**

A. The best prevention is early diagnosis by yearly mammograms, breast self-exams each month, and yearly physical exams by a physician who is skilled in performing breast exams. Dietary changes may be helpful to some degree, but they are not as important as early diagnosis.

Q. **Does exposure to radiation increase the chance of developing breast cancer?**

A. Some studies of atomic bomb survivors indicate an increase in the incidence of breast cancer 10 to 15 years after the radiation. Additional studies of women who have received radiation treatments for tuberculosis also reflected an increase in cancer. This much we do know: The younger a woman is at the time she receives radiation, the greater her chances of developing breast cancer when she gets older. However, if a woman is past the age of 40 when she receives radiation, there does not seem to be an increase in the odds. One important fact to remember: the amount of radiation one receives during a routine mammogram is far less than the amount of radiation one is exposed to in an atomic blast or even with X-ray treatment of breast cancer.

Q. **What is the probability of a female dying of breast cancer?**

A. The average lifetime risk of dying from breast cancer is about 3.6 percent. The following data was taken from CA, a cancer journal for clinicians in 1985:

PROBABILITY OF DYING FROM BREAST CANCER

Period of time	*White women*	*Black women*
Age 20		
within 10 years	0.00	0.02
within 20 years	0.09	0.15
eventually	3.05	3.11
Age 35		
within 10 years	0.14	0.21
within 20 years	0.56	0.72
eventually	3.56	2.98
Age 50		
within 10 years	0.33	0.35
within 20 years	1.04	2.14
eventually	2.75	2.14
Age 65		
within 10 years	0.43	0.26
within 20 years	1.01	0.78
eventually	1.53	1.14

Q. **Does obesity have any adverse effect on the development of breast cancer?**

A. Yes. Several studies indicate that obesity can be harmful for women from postmenopausal age to 70 years of age. In general, women of postmenopausal age who weigh approximately 40 percent more than the ideal body weight run an increased risk of developing breast cancer. It has been suggested that since fat cells can produce estrogen, this higher rate of estrogen in the blood stream of obese women might be related to the higher incidence of breast cancer. Also, obese women consume more fat calories, and increased fat calories might be carcinogenic to the breast cells. Studies also indicate that obese women who are more than 150 pounds overweight are subject to a reduced five year survival from other diseases. But there is good news! Most studies indicate obesity does not have any adverse effects on women of premenopausal age. Obese women in this age bracket tend to have less breast lumps and less breast pain than women who are lean and slim. As a woman approaches menopause, it is important for her to attain and maintain the ideal body weight. Not only will the lack of excess weight decrease the risk of breast cancer, it will also decrease the risk of hypertension, heart disease, diabetes and many other ailments.

Q. **Do large breasts affect my risk of developing breast cancer?**

A. No, they do not, provided there is no family history of breast cancer and previous breast biopsy tissue has not demonstrated any proliferative changes, that is, increased numbers of cells in the breast ducts. Large breasts and a family history of breast cancer, or proliferative changes on previous breast biopsies, does increase the risk of cancer in large breasted women more than small breasted women. Women who have a history of breast cancer in their family should be aware that their risk of developing breast cancer increases at a rate of 1.6. In large-breasted women, this rate is 2.7.

Q. **There is a history of breast cancer in my family. What percentage of breast cancer is genetic or hereditary?**

A. Sporadic breast cancer that is unrelated to any genetic factors accounts for 80 percent to 85 percent of all breast cancer cases.When dominant genes that cause cancer in premenstrual women are passed to a daughter, they account for only 5 percent to 10 percent of all cancer cases. A genetic tendency called familial cancer accounts for about 15 percent of all cancer cases.

Q. **My mother and sister developed breast cancer in their forties, which suggests I may have hereditary breast cancer. Will having a full term baby before I reach my twentieth birthday decrease my risk of developing breast cancer?**

A. Some studies indicate that, with hereditary-type cancer, having an early pregnancy provides no protective effect.

Q. **Does an abortion or a miscarriage at a young age (under 25) decrease or increase the risk of developing breast cancer later in life?**

A. Some studies suggest there is a slight increase in the risk of developing breast cancer if a pregnancy terminates in either an abortion or miscarriage. In order to decrease the risk of developing cancer, the pregnancy must be a term birth or at least reach the last few weeks of the third trimester. When a pregnancy reaches a term birth, the stem cells—cells that transform and become mature normal breast gland cells—become resistant to outside cancer-causing environmental factors (carcinogens). The breast, from the birth forward, becomes more resistant to outside environmental carcinogens.

Q. **Does an early age of menarche (date of first menstruation) affect the risk of developing breast cancer?**

A. Yes, if the age of menarche is 12 years or younger, the relative risk is increased to approximately 1.5. We do not know why, but one theory suggests that stem cells in the breast which grow into mature breast tissue are exposed to outside cancer-producing factors longer (before the first pregnancy). Once the first pregnancy has been achieved, these stem cells become more resistant to the external carcinogens in the environment.

Q. **What effect does the age of menopause have on breast cancer risk?**

A. In general, the older a woman is at menopause the greater her chance of developing breast cancer. Women who menstruate after the age of 55 appear to face the greatest risk, with an increase in the relative risk to about 2.0.

Q. **Does having children affect the incidence or risk of developing breast cancer?**

A. Yes! The younger a woman is at the time of a full term birth, the less risk there is of developing breast cancer. Women who have a child before age 20 enjoy the lowest risk. The risk doesn't decrease appreciably with the birth of more than one child unless the additional term babies are born before the woman reaches 25. Waiting to have the first term baby until age 30 increases the chance of breast cancer to twice that of women who have a baby before age 20. Having the first term baby after age 35 raises the risk of breast cancer more than if a woman remains childless.

Q. **What is meant by relative risk of developing breast cancer?**

A. Relative risk is an equation that measures the increased or decreased chance of one's developing breast cancer compared to other people. Math equation is:

$$\textbf{\textit{The Relative Risk}} = \frac{\dfrac{\textit{Number with cancer among exposed group}}{\textit{Number in exposed group}}}{\dfrac{\textit{Number with cancer among unexposed group}}{\textit{Number in unexposed group}}}$$

An example: If a woman's relative risk is 1.0, it means she has no risk factor for breast cancer, and her lifetime risk is only 3.3 percent, according to a paper by Dr. Newell in the *Journal of Cancer.* If another woman has a relative risk of 1.5 because of something in her background, then her risk of developing breast cancer is 1.5 multiplied by 3.3 percent, giving that woman a 4.95 percent chance of developing breast cancer in her lifetime.

Q. **Please list for me some of the risk factors for breast cancer.**

A.

- Early menarche
- Late menopause
- Nulliparous (no children)
- First born child after age 30
- Being overweight, especially after menopause
- Increasing age
- Breast cancer in primary relative (mother or sister or maternal aunt), especially if the onset was premenopausal

Q. **Is the incidence of breast cancer increasing?**

A. Yes. Unfortunately, it is increasing at a rate of at least 1.4 percent per year in the United States.

Q. **What is the lifetime risk of dying from breast cancer?**

A. Approximately 3.6 percent.

Q. **How many women will die from breast cancer in 1994?**

A. Approximately 48,000 are predicted. Only lung cancer will cause more cancer deaths.

Q. **My mother and sister developed breast cancer while in their late thirties. Does this increase my chances of developing breast cancer?**

A. If a woman has a mother and a sister or a mother and a maternal grandmother with premenopausal breast cancer, her lifetime risk will be approximately 1 in 3. If the disease is bilateral (in both breasts) in either relative, the risk increases to approximately 1 in 2.

Q. About what percentage of women get breast cancer in their twenties and thirties?

A. Of all the women who develop breast cancer, about 2 percent are in their twenties and 6 percent are less than 40 years of age.

Q. My mother developed breast cancer when she was postmenopausal. Does that increase my risk of breast cancer?

A. Slightly. A postmenopausal mother who develops breast cancer will increase the relative lifetime risk of her daughter developing breast cancer to approximately 1.8.

Q. Fact or fiction? Tall women develop more breast cancer.

A. Some studies indicate a very small increase in cancer risk in tall women in the U.S. Studies between different countries show that countries with taller women have a higher rate of breast cancer. This difference between countries is believed to be due to better nutrition.

Q. Does having my first child at age 38 decrease my chance of developing breast cancer as compared to not having any children at all?

A. Not necessarily. A childless woman has about the same risk of breast cancer as a woman who has her first birth at age 30. Women who have a first child in their late thirties have a slightly higher risk of developing breast cancer than if they remain childless.

Q. **Does being lean affect the chance of developing breast cancer?**

A. At different stages of your life, yes. Women who are lean and premenopausal have an increased relative risk of approximately 1.4. After menopause, obesity increases the relative risk to approximately 1.5, and leanness becomes an advantage instead of a disadvantage.

Q. **Does taking birth control pills increase my risk of breast cancer?**

A. No. Most studies reflect no relationship between birth control pills and breast cancer, except with two sub-groups of women. Sub-group one is women who use birth control pills around the time of menopause and especially between the age of 51 to 55; these women show a significantly increased risk. The other sub-group is women who use birth control pills at an early age and for a long duration before their first pregnancy. These women who delay their first pregnancy have a slight increase in the relative risk of breast cancer. Note that these sub-group studies are not conclusive at this time.

Q. **Does having my ovaries removed (an oophorectomy) affect my chance of developing breast cancer?**

A. Having an oophorectomy by age 35 decreases your risk of developing breast cancer to approximately one-half the relative risk. Having an oophorectomy in the mid-forties will decrease the relative risk to approximately 0.8. If you take estrogen replacement, the risk will be about the same as if the oophorectomy was never performed.

Q. **My mother developed breast cancer at age 48. Does taking birth control pills increase my chance of developing breast cancer more because my mother developed breast cancer?**

A. No. Your risk is no greater than that of any woman who has a first degree relative with breast cancer.

Q. **Does taking hormones after menopause increase my risk of developing breast cancer?**

A. No. Most studies of estrogen use after menopause have shown essentially no increase in breast cancer. However, some recent studies indicated a possible increased risk, though small, in the early months of use. This slightly increased risk could be a result of estrogen stimulating the growth of a tumor already present in the breast. The risk seems to disappear after stopping the hormones for one year. It is interesting to note that the Nurses' Health Study shows that women who were diagnosed with breast cancer while taking hormones had lower mortality from the cancer than women who were found to have cancer and were *not* taking hormones.

Adding progestin (Provera) to postmenopausal therapy has not been adequately evaluated to determine if the progestins are helpful in reducing breast cancer.

All women should know that taking postmenopausal hormones usually improves the quality of life by keeping the sexual organs, bones, skin, and arteries younger.

Q. **Does breast-feeding increase or decrease my chance of developing breast cancer?**

A. Past studies that have adjusted for the multiple factors of breast cancer, especially age at first birth, do not suggest any protective effect. A new study, however, suggests otherwise. The January 1994 *New England Journal of Medicine* reported a new large study that demonstrated that women who breast-feed four or more months had less premenopausal breast cancer; but it indicated no effect on the rate of postmenopausal breast cancer. The authors predicted that if all women breast-feed 24 months or longer, the incidence of breast cancer could be reduced up to 25 percent, especially if women began breast-feeding at a younger age.

Q. **I have heard that women in higher socio-economic classes have a 50 percent greater chance of developing breast cancer than those women in lower socio-economic classes. Is this true?**

A. Yes. Women in higher socio-economic classes do have a higher incidence of breast cancer. Some of the increased rate is probably related to the late age of first birth, but when one adjusts for ages at first birth, there is still a higher rate for women in higher socio-economic groups.

Q. **Will eating less fat decrease my chance of developing breast cancer?**

A. The differences in the breast cancer rate between different countries that have different amounts of fat in the diet have fueled the argument that the increased fat in the American diet may contribute to breast cancer. Animal studies indicate that a high fat diet and a carcinogen added to the diet will increase the incidence of breast cancer. Some believe that the caloric surplus of these studies has more effect than the percentage of calories derived from fat.

Groups of Americans who are studied for different amounts of fat in their diet do not indicate any difference in breast cancer risk. The largest study was the Nurses' Health Study which showed that nurses who had 44 percent of their calories from fat (a highly undesirable amount) had a slightly less than average risk of developing breast cancer.

It is possible that the fat in the diet early in life may explain the international difference in breast cancer rate based on fat consumption. In other words, a high fat diet may affect the stem cells in the breast at an early age and before the first term pregnancy is delivered.

Q. Do viruses cause breast cancers?

A. Viruses have been shown to cause breast cancer in monkeys and mice, but so far, no virus has conclusively been shown to cause human breast cancers. However, viral particles similar to the animal virus have been found in human milk. Women that have a strong family history of breast cancer have a much higher incidence of these viral particles being found in their breast milk.

Q. Has the survival rate for breast cancer improved over the years?

A. The five year survival has improved.

Year 1961 .... 63% survival 5 years
Year 1971 .... 68% survival 5 years
Year 1984 .... 78% survival 5 years

Q. I had a breast biopsy about five years ago. Does having a previous breast biopsy increase my risk of developing breast cancer?

A. Cutting into the breast does not cause breast cancer. If your previous breast biopsy showed that you had normal breast tissue or normal fibrocystic changes ***(See Chapter 7)***, your chance of developing breast cancer is not increased. If your breast biopsy showed abnormal changes, your chance of cancer would be increased.

Q. Will participating in sports or doing vigorous physical activity decrease my daughter's chances of developing breast cancer?

A. Young women athletes have a slight reduction in their lifetime risk of developing breast cancer. The reason for this is unknown, but some feel that the delay in menarche or non-ovulating menstrual cycles in athletes may account for the protective effect.

Q. **Does drinking alcohol affect the chance of developing breast cancer?**

A. Most studies have shown an increase in breast cancer with alcohol consumption. The Nurses' Health Study demonstrated an increase of the relative risk to 1.3 with only one drink per day. When the many studies are evaluated, there is continued increase in cancer with the increase in alcohol consumption. Why alcohol causes the cancer risk to increase is not known. Some epidemiologists feel that the adverse effect of alcohol is especially significant in women who drank alcohol before the age of thirty. Alcohol seems to be an independent factor and could account for at least 10 percent of all breast cancer cases.

Q. **Does smoking affect my risk of breast cancer?**

A. Smokers have an earlier menopause and reduced secretion of estrogens in their urine, yet there is no conclusive evidence that smoking has any effect on the incidence of breast cancer.

Q. **Does taking Vitamin A help prevent breast cancer?**

A. Vitamin A is known to maintain the health of skin cells. Some of the retinoids (chemicals similar to Vitamin A) have been shown to have a protective effect on breast cells as well. In laboratory experiments using animals, retinoids prevented breast cancer. However, most retinoids are quite toxic and are not recommended for human use. In Italy, a study is currently under way to determine if retinoids can be helpful to humans.

Q. **Does selenium (a trace mineral) protect one from breast cancer?**

A. Studies have shown selenium to have a protective effect on animals when a carcinogen (cancer-causing substance) is given to them. In addition, some epidemiologic studies suggest a lower cancer rate in regions having a high selenium content in the soil. A prospective study of the amount of selenium in the toe nail clippings of the Nurses' Health Study did not show any helpful effect of selenium. The conclusion is this: selenium is a toxic metal if taken in large quantities, and any helpful effect of adding extra selenium to one's diet has not been resolved.

Q. **If my mother breast-fed me, am I less likely to develop breast cancer?**

A. Unfortunately, the answer to this question is not known at this time.

Q. **What are the risk factors for developing breast cancer, and which ones are more important?**

A. **MAJOR FACTORS increasing risk:**

- age
- family history of breast cancer
- abnormal (proliferative) changes in breast biopsy tissue

MINOR FACTORS increasing risks:

- menarche before age 12
- no children before age 30
- menopause after age 50
- high socio-economic status
- high-fat diet, alcohol use
- increased body weight and height
- ionizing radiation as a child (moderate dose)
- not breast-feeding

Q. **What criteria are used to calculate the possibility of hereditary breast cancer, the type of cancer that makes up 5 percent of all breast cancers?**

A. The following criteria generally have to be met:

- two or more first degree relatives, such as sisters or a mother
- cancer in premenopausal relative, especially bilateral cancer
- cancer in several generations

Q. **I now have breast cancer, so what is the chance of my relatives developing breast cancer?**

A. Here are some estimates calculated from M.D. Anderson Hospital based on their patient data. (These numbers may be higher than the actual risk because of the statistical method used to compute risk.)

You the patient	***Risk to sisters, mothers and daughters compared to controls relative risk increase***
Premenopausal	*3.1*
Postmenopausal	*1.5*
Bilateral	*5.4*
Unilateral	*1.3*
Premenopausal & Bilateral	*8.8*
Premenopausal & Unilateral	*1.8*
Postmenopausal & Bilateral	*4.0*
Postmenopausal and Unilateral	*1.2*

Q. **I have heard about a gene that causes breast cancer. What about this?**

A. There is a gene on the 17th chromosome called BRCA1. This genetic abnormality was discovered in 1990. If a woman has BRAC1, her chances of developing breast cancer by the age of 90 are about 85 percent. About one in every 300 women carry this abnormal gene. It is believed to cause about 5 percent of all breast cancer. Women who have this gene also have a higher chance of developing ovarian cancer and cancer of both breasts.

Q. **Can I find out if I am a carrier of a defect on chromosome 17 that will increase my chance of breast cancer?**

A. Commercial testing for the BRCA1 gene is not available at this time. It is hoped that in the next several years genetic analysis will be available.

Q. **What percentage of hereditary breast cancer is from BRCA1?**

A. Presently, it is believed that about 45 percent of all hereditary breast cancer is the result of an abnormality of the BRCA1 gene on chromosome 17.

Q. **If I find out that I carry the BRCA1 gene, what will happen to my insurance?**

A. At present, there are many social, ethical, and privacy issues which are not known.

Q. **What are my chances of developing breast cancer based on my relative having breast cancer?**

A. One study called the CASH Study gives the following relative risks:

No family history	1
Mother or sister	2.3
Grandmother or aunt	1.5
Mother and sister	up to 14

Q. **Why does breast cancer cluster in some families?**

A. There are many factors, some of which are felt to be culturally shared risk factors, such as: 1) late childbirth; 2) common environmental factors, i.e., diet; and 3) genetic similarities and susceptibility.

Q. **If I have hereditary breast cancer in my family, will I decrease my chance of breast cancer if I have children at a young age?**

A. It seems that having children at an early age does not have any protective effect on women with hereditary breast cancer.

Q. **Is there any drug that I can take to decrease my chance of developing breast cancer?**

A. Tamoxifen taken daily has been shown to decrease the chance of breast cancer in rats. It is presently in clinical investigation in both the United States and Great Britain to determine if it will reduce the rate of cancer among women who are at high risk of developing breast cancer. This investigation is just beginning, and as many as 10 to 15 years may be needed to determine if the drug is effective. At this time, the FDA has not approved the use of tamoxifen to decrease the risk of cancer in women who have not developed breast cancer. Also, Tamoxifen is not without small potential risks. Its use has been linked to heart disease, cataracts, liver cancer and uterine cancer.

Q. **If a woman has a father who develops breast cancer, is she at greater risk of developing breast cancer?**

A. Breast cancer in males is quite rare and no definite answer is known at this time. This we do know: The gene to develop hereditary cancer is not sex determined. A father has a 50 percent chance of passing the gene to his daughters.

Q. **What are the five most common cancers in women, and the five most common cancers leading to death in women?**

A. Excluding basal and squamous skin cancers, the American Cancer Society, in *Cancer Journal for Clinicians*, gives the following statistics:

Cancer incidence by site, estimated for 1993

Site	Percent
Breast	*32%*
Colon and Rectum	*13%*
Lung	*12%*
Uterus	*8%*
Leukemia & Lymphoma	*6%*

Cancer deaths by site, estimated for 1993

Site	Percent
Lung	*22%*
Breast	*18%*
Colon & Rectum	*11%*
Leukemia & Lymphoma	*8%*
Pancreas	*5%*

Chapter Three

CANCER DETECTION

Q&A At what age should a woman begin mammograms?

A woman without known increased risk factors should have a baseline mammogram between the ages of 35 and 40. If one of her first degree relatives, a mother or sister or aunt, has had breast cancer after menopause, she should begin having mammograms closer to age 35. However, if the relative's cancer was found *before* menopause, the patient's own risk is greater. Mammograms and BSE (breast self-exam) should begin five to ten years before the age of cancer detection in the relative.

Q. **Is a mammogram alone able to find all breast cancers?**

A. No. There is no single perfect medical test that will detect all breast cancers. Most, but not all, cancers can be detected earlier by a mammogram than by a physical exam; however, normal dense glandular tissue seen on the mammogram can hide cancers. In fact, approximately 10 percent of cancers will be invisible on a mammogram but will be felt on a physical examination or be discovered on BSE. This is why mammography should be used in combination with a physical examination by a physician. If there is a lump or a question of one, consult a surgeon, even if the mammogram is negative. *This cannot be stressed too strongly.*

Q. **How often should a woman have a mammogram?**

A. Once a year is best. For women in their forties, every one or two years is the official recommendation of the American Cancer Society and other organizations in this country; for women 50 and over, a mammogram every year.

Cancer in young women typically grows faster than in older women, so some countries, such as Sweden, recommend mammography every twelve months for women under 50. A two-year interval between mammograms is too long and could result in potentially curable cancers becoming larger and therefore lethal during the second year.

Q. **If a lump is discovered between mammograms, what should be done and when?**

A. First, go see your doctor. This possible lump can be investigated in may different ways, depending on what your doctor thinks after the examination. It might be a liquid cyst which can be easily drained by a needle, a simple procedure called aspiration. Your doctor may request you to get a diagnostic mammogram and a breast sonogram (ultrasound). Or you may be sent to a surgeon for consideration of a biopsy. The most important point is this: Don't wait. Act now. A negative mammogram six months earlier does not eliminate the possibility of cancer. This is why monthly breast self-examination (BSE) is encouraged and taught in most breast centers and doctors' offices.

Q. **Is it safe to have mammography and sonography (ultrasound) of the breast during pregnancy?**

A. Safe, yes. During mammography the fetus is exposed to very little radiation if a shield is used over the abdomen, and sonography has no risk whatsoever. Understand, however, that mammography and sonography are not as accurate during pregnancy because increased growth of blood vessels and water content in the breast can alter and obscure the view of breast tissue.

Q. **How does an ultrasound evaluate the breast?**

A. A radiologist will request an ultrasound for additional evaluation if something suspicious appears on the mammogram. For instance, ultrasound is used to help evaluate masses that are palpable or visible on a mammogram. While mammograms cannot reveal if a lesion is solid or cystic, an ultrasound can, and this information determines treatment. If the ultrasound reveals that the mass is cystic, it is unlikely it will need to be biopsied.

Ultrasound can also be used to aid in fine-needle aspiration biopsies on nonpalpable lesions and for preoperative localizations that cannot be seen by mammography. If a woman has a choice of either mammography or ultrasound, it is advisable to select the more sensitive mammography. Ultrasound will only pick up about 40 percent of all cancers when used alone.

Q. **What is the incidence of breast cancer discovered during pregnancy?**

A. We're not really sure. Two different studies reflect different results. One study indicates breast cancer to be as high as one in every 1,500 pregnancies, while another study concludes there is only one case of breast cancer in every 3,000 pregnancies.

Q. **At what age should monthly breast self-examination begin?**

A. Years before you are likely to begin mammograms, you have a risk for breast cancer. This risk is statistically very small if you are in your twenties and thirties, but if you do develop a cancer then, a cure is possible only during a very brief period of time and depends on prompt action.

So, start the self exams in your twenties. If you have any questions about your monthly exam, do not ignore them. See your doctor immediately.

Q. **Are mammograms useful at all ages?**

A. No. During adolescence and in the early twenties, the breast is composed of dense glandular tissue which is difficult to penetrate with X-rays. If a lump is discovered, it should of course be investigated, and the radiologist will probably use ultrasound first, possibly followed by a mammogram. After age thirty, breast tissue density tends to decrease somewhat and mammography becomes the primary choice, with ultrasound being used as a possible follow-up.

Q. **How accurate is mammography if I have implants? Will it damage my implants?**

A. Implants will obscure some of the tissue on the standard mammogram views, so extra views, called Eklund views, named after the radiologist who developed the technique, will also be done.

Standard views will be taken to show the implants and some tissue above, below, and on either side of the implant. Then the technologist pulls the breast forward and holds the implant back out of the view as she applies the compression. In this way, the breast is properly compressed for viewing and is seen without the implant.

The amount of breast tissue visualized with the Eklund views is almost the same as if there were no implants, so accuracy is only slightly compromised in women with implants. Implants are tested before insertion and can safely withstand forces much greater than those generated during mammography, so the exam is safe.

Q. **I've heard women say mammograms are painful. Is this always true?**

A. No. Thanks to experienced technologists, the majority of women do not report pain with mammograms; however, some women do find the procedure uncomfortable. This discomfort is temporary and can be reduced by less compression. But less compression can result in films that are too "light," which means there was not enough compression to allow good X-ray penetration through the breast, and the technologist will have to repeat the procedure.

If you are one of the women who finds mammograms painful, following a few simple precautions will help. Cut back on caffeine a few days before your mammogram, and schedule the procedure during the first half of your menstrual cycle when the tissue is less sensitive.

If your mammogram was painful last year, tell the technologist. She may reduce the compression force to a more tolerable level. While the resulting films could be slightly underpenetrated, it is far better to have yearly mammograms that are slightly underpenetrated than to have no mammograms at all. In order to discover breast cancer early, these tests will need to be done throughout your life.

Q. **What is the significance of calcification on a mammogram?**

A. Most breast calcifications are benign. They occur in the glands of the breast where the milk is secreted and give a distinctive appearance, shaped like fluid in the bottom of a teacup. Others are in blood vessels, and some are found in the glands of the skin.

Calcifications that warrant concern are those that occur in the small ducts of the breast that lead away from the glands or lobules: these calcifications may be due to cancer cells. At this stage, with calcification present but no lump, surgical removal often accomplishes a cure.

Q. **If a mammogram has microcalcifications that look like grains of salt, how many specks of calcium are necessary to have a malignancy if no mass is seen on the mammogram?**

A. It is not only the number of calcifications but also the shape and the density that is important in arriving at a diagnosis. If more than one or two calcifications are located in a very small volume of tissue, there is a good chance that the radiologist will order magnification views in order to see the calcification more clearly. Sometimes only two or three calcifications can indicate a malignancy if no mass is present, but usually there will be more than five.

Q. **Does taking calcium tablets to help my bones cause me to get calcium on my mammogram?**

A. There is no evidence that taking extra calcium in a diet causes calcium in the breast. Also, the calcium doesn't cause the cancer. Malignant calcifications are the result of cancer cells that have outgrown their blood supply and died.

Q. **What are magnification views and spot views?**

A. If the initial screening mammogram views reveal calcification, the radiologist may order special views that magnify the calcium particles, enlarging them so that the shape, density, and number of particles can be better seen. This information is used to determine the need for a biopsy. Spot views are extra views of just one area of a breast that looked somewhat suspicious on the first screening films. If a lump or nodule is truly present, it will look the same in size and shape on the new "spot" film. If the suspected abnormality is nothing more than normal glands superimposed on each other, the extra views show this clearly.

Q. **If a new solid mass is found on a mammogram, what should be done? Biopsy? Follow-up mammogram in six months?**

A. The decision to wait six months or to immediately undergo a biopsy is a serious one and should be made with caution.

Even a small, smooth nodule which is solid (proven by ultrasound exam) has a chance of malignancy. If it is not smooth, the odds of it being malignant increase. A mass having a very irregular surface with tiny sticker-like spikes around the border is almost certainly cancerous.

A biopsy is usually recommended for any new solid nodule. Fortunately, open surgical biopsy with general anesthesia poses very little risk, and core biopsy using local anesthesia has even less risk and cost; however, waiting six months for a follow-up mammogram after the discovery of a new solid mass risks allowing a small cancer to grow and spread beyond the breast.

Q. **When did doctors start performing mammograms and believe they could be effective in detecting cancer?**

A. Mammogram was first described in 1913 by a German surgeon. In the United States, Dr. Robert Egan established a technique for mammogram in the 1950s. Mammography use has grown steadily since the 1960s, when studies started to demonstrate that early detection of breast cancers using mammograms extended women's lives.

Q. **Why should I have a mammogram?**

A. Mammograms can detect breast cancer before it becomes a palpable lump. This is important because small breast tumors are more curable since they are less likely to have spread (metastasized).

Q. **Is there more than one type of mammogram?**

A. In 1972, two new types of mammograms were introduced which decreased the amount of radiation required. One type utilizes X-ray film and is called film-screen mammography. The other type is called Xeromammography, which uses special Xerox paper.

Q. Which type of mammography technique has greater accuracy?

A. Most studies show neither technique has significant difference in accuracy.

Q. Which technique of taking mammograms is most widely used?

A. Film-screen mammography is more widely used because the equipment required is less expensive. In 1989, the Xerox corporation discontinued manufacturing the special X-ray equipment for the Xerox process of taking mammograms, although existing equipment is still in use and the paper is still being manufactured.

Q. Which mammography technique offers the least radiation?

A. Film-screen mammography gives the least radiation for a two-view examination. Approximately 0.05 rad to 0.1 rad is delivered by film-screen mammography; 0.13 rad to 0.26 rad is delivered by Xeromammography, depending on the different techniques for each type of X-ray. Don't forget that a person receives more radiation than this when flying in an airplane between Dallas and Denver.

Q. During a mammogram, why does the technician have to squeeze my breasts and compress them so firmly?

A. Compressing the breast improves the quality of the mammogram in several ways: 1) it causes uniform thickness and allows comparison of different parts of each breast; 2) it brings the breast structures closer to the X-ray film, making them sharper; 3) less radiation is required to penetrate the tissue of a thin, compressed breast; and 4) more breast tissue is exposed to the film.

Q. **How does a physician know if a mass seen in a mammogram is benign or malignant?**

A. Masses that have a smooth border are usually benign. If the mass is less than half an inch in size and is smooth, the chances of it being benign are great. A mass that has an irregular border has approximately a 10 percent to 50 percent chance of being malignant. A mass that has a stellate border (having sticker-like spikes) is malignant over 75 percent of the time.

Q. **Has the use of mammography changed the chance of survival of breast cancer?**

A. Absolutely. According to studies, women who had a nonpalpable cancer discovered on mammography and then underwent appropriate treatment have a longer survival than women with breast cancer who have not had routine mammography.

Q. **How accurate are mammograms, and what percent of cancers do they miss?**

A. Mammography misses approximately 10 percent to 15 percent of breast cancers. The good news is that they accurately detect 85 percent to 90 percent of all breast cancers.

Q. **Why do mammograms not detect all breast cancers?**

A. Dense breast tissue is why mammograms may miss cancers. There simply is not enough difference between a dense cancer and dense breast tissue to determine any abnormality. Density of the breast is why mammograms for women in their 30s and 40s fail to detect more cancers in these ages than at older ages. Mammographic technique and a radiologist's skill are much less of a factor.

Q. **If all U.S. women followed the recommended guidelines for screening mammography, how much would the mortality from breast cancer be decreased?**

A. It is estimated that the mortality from breast cancer would be reduced at least 30 percent to 40 percent if all U. S. women followed the Cancer Society's guidelines for routine screening mammography.

Q. **If a mass is seen on a mammogram, what characteristics will indicate that the mass should be biopsied?**

A. The contour of a mass helps determine if it is malignant. If the contour is smooth, this indicates that cell growth is controlled, so the likelihood of malignancy is low. If the contour is irregular or lobulated, indicating cellular growth that is uncontrolled, the chance of malignancy is greater. If the margins are blurred or spike-like, the cellular growth is more rapid and uncontrolled.

Q. **About how many women in the United States have had a mammogram?**

A. About 30 percent of all women that should have a mammogram have had at least one mammogram in their life. Far fewer women have a yearly mammogram, but the exact percentage is not known.

Q. **Have radiologists standardized the way mammogram reports are reported?**

A. Yes. In 1992, the American College of Radiology attempted to standardize five different categories for reporting the possibility of a mammogram showing a malignant finding.

Category 0—No radiographic findings of a malignancy. This category may include a cyst.

Category 1—Benign findings with no radiographic evidence of malignancy.

This category could include a fibroadenoma or a mass that has been stable for greater than 2 years so was felt to be benign.

Category 2—Indeterminate findings, probably benign.

This category means that on a routine mammogram there are new findings which have some possibility of malignancy and need follow up with a breast surgeon or further mammographic studies. If a lesion is in this category, the chance of malignancy is 5-10 percent.

Category 3—Indeterminate findings, possibly malignant.

This category means that there is a finding mammographically which has approximately a 50 percent chance of being malignant.

Category 4—Probably malignant.

This category means that the chance of the findings seen on the mammogram have at least a 75 percent chance of being malignant.

The American College of Radiology hopes that by using these new categories more useful information will be obtained so that the patient and her doctor can make a correct decision regarding the need for a biopsy.

Q. **How important are breast self-exams (BSE)?**

A. Most cancerous lumps are found by women examining their own breasts. Some studies have shown that women who practice BSE have cancers that are smaller when found. Only a woman can learn all the subtle aspects of her own breasts so she can prevent needless biopsies of the normal lumpiness of her breasts.

Q. **When should I do a breast self-exam?**

A. The best time is about one week after menstruation stops, because the breasts are less engorged and tender. If one has stopped menstruating because of age or surgical removal of the ovaries, picking a day around the first of each month is recommended.

Q. **How do I do a breast self-exam?**

A. **Step 1:** Visually inspect the breast in front of a mirror from three different positions—with the arms in the overhead position, arms at the side, and arms placed on the hips. Check for skin retraction or dimpling, nipple changes such as retraction, discharge, or scaling of the skin, and compare the breasts for shape, lumps, and redness of the skin. **Step 2:** Palpate the breasts. This is best done while you are lying down because it makes the breasts thinner, making any abnormalities easier to feel. *All* areas of the breast must be examined—this is especially important. With the pads of the fingers (because they are more sensitive than the fingertips), use small circular motions to examine the opposite breast. Applying light, gentle pressure, examine the more superficial tissue of the breast. Increase the pressure to evaluate deeper portions of the breast. You are looking for solitary lumps that are hard, irregular, and are not tender. Symmetrical findings are usually benign. If your breast self-exam indicates a new difference in the tissue between the two breasts, a difference you did not notice during your last breast self-exam, see your doctor for a professional exam.

It is not recommended that you squeeze your nipples during breast self-exam because this can cause the nipples to express normal fluid (of a greenish or milky color) and can also irritate the nipples, causing them to produce more fluid. Only in the case of a spontaneous discharge or a bloody discharge from the nipple do you need to see a physician.

Q. **My gynecologist used to do thermography on my breasts to detect cancer. Why does he no longer do this study?**

A. Thermography was started in the 1950s when it was discovered that breast cancers caused a rise in the skin temperature over the cancer. It is now determined that the sensitivity of this study is less than 50 percent, so it is no longer used.

Q. **My girlfriend used to get light scanning of her breasts for cancer detection. Should I ask for this study?**

A. Light scanning of the breast has been used because it was found that the increased blood in breast cancers would absorb more light than normal breast tissue. The sensitivity of this study is only about half the sensitivity of mammograms, so it is seldom performed.

Q. **Approximately what percentage of women that receive a breast biopsy based on a mammogram abnormality will have cancer?**

A. This can vary greatly depending on the diagnostic team involved, but in general, one cancer should be detected for every three to four women who are biopsied. However, a more important statistic to look at in any breast screening practice is whether small, potentially curable cancers are being detected at a significant rate. In other words, is their mammography sensitive at detecting small cancers? What percentage of the cancers detected are under two-thirds of an inch in size and have not yet spread to the lymph nodes?

Q. **If I have a screening mammography exam, what are my chances that they will find something wrong?**

A. This question is difficult to answer because it depends on one's age, with younger patients having a lower incidence of breast cancer, but it is possible to estimate. Assuming a screening van came to a large company and

100 women had mammograms, the results would be approximately these: 90 percent would be interpreted as normal; 5–10 percent would require repeat special views or ultrasound; 1–2 percent would require biopsy of suspicious mammogram findings.

Q. **What are the chances of the different contours of a mass seen on a mammogram being malignant?**

A. An estimate of a mass being malignant is as follows: smooth border—less than 5 percent malignant; irregular border—10 percent to 50 percent malignant; stellate (spiked) border—75 percent to 80 percent malignant.

Q. **My friend's mammogram cost about twice as much as mine. She said she had eight X-rays and I only had four X-rays. Can you explain this?**

A. First, costs of mammography vary from one center to the next. The busier mammography institutions usually have a lower-priced "screening" study for women without lumps or special symptoms such as discharge. This screening study consists of two films of each breast and the radiologist carefully interprets them later, usually the next day. Reading them immediately would increase the time and create delays for everyone. Remember, what matters is not how fast your radiologist reads the films, it is how accurately.

If you have a lump, or if you just do not want any chance of being recalled at a later day, you will receive a "diagnostic" mammogram, which is studied and interpreted while you are there. This takes longer, but any additional views and ultrasound can be done if needed while you are present at the appointment. A diagnostic mammogram usually costs more than a screening mammogram.

For most women, the screening study is usually the

best choice, since 90 percent of the time the screening will be clear and will not require a call back for special views.

Q. **What is the main use of MRI (magnetic resonance imaging)?**

A. Probably the main use for MRI is to detect silicone. MRI is used to determine if there is a leak of an implant or if a mass has formed from the silicone.

Q. **Should MRI be used instead of conventional mammography?**

A. So far, no studies indicate that screening MRI would be superior to conventional X-ray mammography. Presently, the least expensive MRI is still ten times the cost of conventional mammography. Many insurance companies feel MRI is experimental and do not pay for it.

Q. **As technology improves, can we expect to see more use of MRI in the detection of breast cancer in the future?**

A. Yes. In the future, scientists hope that MRI will be able to do two things: 1) decrease the number of biopsies needed by being more exact than the mammogram; and 2) determine if there is any additional cancer in the breast that needs to be surgically removed to prevent a recurrence after a lumpectomy.

Q. **On my recent mammogram, something was discovered that the radiologist was concerned about, so the radiologist wanted me to return in four to six months for a follow-up mammogram. What should I do?**

A. Some well-respected radiologists recommend follow-up mammographic exams rather than immediate surgery for probable benign lesions. With the cost consciousness of present medicine this may be recommended more frequently in the future. If, however, only a screening mammogram has been done and the recommendation is a follow-up in six months, it would be far better to immediately investigate further with additional special mammograms (spot views) and possibly sonography. A second opinion from another radiologists may be helpful. The six-month follow-up should only be done for a probable benign abnormality that had been fully worked up with special mammographic views, and it should only be done if the patient fully understands that there are other options, namely immediate open surgical biopsy or core biopsy ***(See Chapter 7)***.

Q. **What percentage of palpable breast lumps will not be seen on mammography?**

A. A study in 1982 demonstrated that 9 percent of palpable breast cancers were not seen on mammograms. This fact makes BSE important, along with the mammogram.

Chapter Four

LUMPS AND CYSTS

Q. How common are breast cysts?

A. Approximately 30 percent of all women develop breast cysts between ages 35 and 50. These cysts usually do not cause them any problems or symptoms. After age 35, the glandular tissue in the breast decreases and cysts develop as a result of the normal aging processes. About 7 percent of women who develop breast cysts see a physician for treatment. Only about 5 percent of cysts occur before age 30 or after age 55.

Q. **Do the number of cysts vary among women?**

A. About half of all women who develop breast cysts have only a single cyst, but one-third of these women will have two to five cysts. A small proportion of women will have more than five cysts.

Q. **Do cysts occur equally in both breasts?**

A. In his textbook, Dr. C. D. Haagensen reports that the left breast is slightly more likely to have a cyst.

Q. **Do cysts change in size?**

A. Serial mammograms and sonograms demonstrate that cysts increase and decrease in size.

Q. **Why do we aspirate cysts?**

A. Cysts are aspirated for five different reasons: 1) to make sure that the mass is indeed a cyst; 2) to relieve the pain of a cyst if it is painful; 3) to improve the accuracy of a mammogram, since a cyst can obscure mammographic findings; 4) to determine if a mass is present after the cyst is aspirated; and 5) to determine if the cyst contains blood.

Q. When do cysts need to be biopsied?

A. Cysts *may* need to be biopsied for the following reasons: 1) if the fluid aspirated from a cyst is bloody, since there is a chance that the cyst may contain a small tumor; 2) if a lump or mass still exists after the cyst has been aspirated; 3) if there is an abnormal sonogram or pneumocystogram showing abnormal tissue inside the cyst suggesting a tumor (a pneumocystogram is when air is injected inside the cyst to help better visualize the cyst lining). In some instances, surgeons remove a cyst if it has recurred three or four times in one breast. Up to one percent of these recurrent cysts may contain tumor cells.

Q. Does the fluid from a cyst need to be examined?

A. The fluid from a cyst contains formless debris from dead cells. Numerous studies show that there is little benefit from evaluating the fluid. Some physicians, however, do favor evaluating the fluid if it is bloody.

Q. Does the color of the fluid in a breast cyst have any significance?

A. In general, the color of the fluid varies with the age of the cyst. In older cysts, the color of the fluid is darker, ranging from dark brown to a greenish gray. Young cysts contain thinner fluid and the color is more straw colored.

Q. Is there any type of cystic fluid that is more likely to indicate cancer?

A. Only bloody fluid suggests the possibility of malignancy. Cystic fluid has been analyzed for electrolytes, proteins, and hormones. There is no conclusive evidence that any special substance other than blood in a cyst predicts the development of breast cancer.

Q. **Are there different types of cysts?**

A. One way cysts have been classified is by determining potassium concentrations in the cyst fluid. Cysts with high potassium values are actively secreting substances into the fluid. Most small cysts, less than one-half inch, have high potassium levels in the fluid.

Q. **Why does a cyst form?**

A. The balance between secretion, outflow, and reabsorption of fluid is disrupted. The ducts draining glandular breast tissue may be replaced with connective tissue, or may become plugged by too many cells in the duct wall; either of these conditions can interfere with the absorption of gland fluids. Cell secretion can also exceed the reabsorption capacity of the glandular tissue. Increased estrogen levels, particularly in postmenopausal women, sometimes increases cyst formation, since estrogen can increase fluid secretion from breast cells in the acini.

Q. **Are different cyst types more likely to recur?**

A. Women with high potassium levels in the cyst fluid tend to develop other cysts. When cysts do recur, they are usually the same type.

Q. **Since I have not had any children, does that make me more likely to develop cysts?**

A. Women without children develop slightly more cysts than women who have given birth.

Q. **Why do some cysts cause pain?**

A. Physicians believe cystic pain is caused by fluid high in potassium leaking into the surrounding tissue. This produces a chemical irritation.

Q. **In what location do cysts occur in the breast?**

A. Approximately 55 percent of all cysts are in the left breast. Two-thirds of all cysts occur in the upper outer quadrant near the armpit.

Q. **What percentage of cysts recur?**

A. Approximately 10 percent to 15 percent of cysts will recur after aspiration. About 50 percent of all women who have a cyst will sometime develop a second cyst somewhere else in the breast.

Q. **What age group is more likely to develop breast cysts?**

A. Cysts are most common in the 35- to 50-year-old age group. Only two to three percent of women less than 30 years of age or above age 55 develop cysts. However, cysts are more common among women on estrogen replacement therapy. If you are taking estrogen and having cyst problems, stopping the estrogen will probably help stop the cysts from recurring.

Q. **Do women who develop breast cysts have abnormal concentrations of hormones?**

A. Women with cysts do not have any hormone imbalance, although some studies have detected high concentrations of hormones in some cysts. The significance of this finding is not known.

Q. **Are there any medications or dietary habits that can prevent cyst formation?**

A. Danazol, which is a weak male hormone, may help decrease the size of cysts and may prevent their recurrence. Danazol, however, can cause a woman to develop facial hair and a change in her voice, so it is not routinely prescribed. Changing your diet to avoid all caffeine has been suggested, although there is no conclusive proof that the avoidance of caffeine intake has any effect in reducing the number of cysts. Stopping the use of caffeine, however, has helped reduce breast pain for many women.

Q. **Does having breast cysts increase the chance of developing breast cancer?**

A. Although there have been many studies on this subject, there is no clear relationship between breast cysts and the development of breast cancer. From these numerous studies, only two or three have found an increased risk of breast cancer. An increased risk was found among women with large (gross) breast cysts who also have a family history of cancer.

Q. **What is fibrocystic disease?**

A. The term fibrocystic disease is inaccurate, since this normal breast condition is not a disease. Normal fibrocystic *changes* occur in breast tissue with each menstrual cycle, and these changes also accompany the natural aging process. As the breasts age, the breast glandular cells and ductal cells die and are replaced with either fibrous tissue or fat tissue. The replacement of the breast tissue in uneven distributions causes the breast to be lumpy. A better name for this normal condition of the breast would be fibrocystic changes.

Q. **How do you know when a change such as a new lump in a fibrocystic breast needs to be evaluated?**

A. Guidelines for seeing a physician for a breast change include the following: 1) changes that do not resolve after one menstrual cycle; 2) breast discomfort that does not disappear after one menstrual cycle; 3) a single breast lump that feels different from other lumps in the breast; 4) discharge from one nipple.

Q. **Does caffeine in coffee and chocolate cause fibrocystic breast changes?**

A. There is no proof that caffeine contributes to lumpiness of the breast. In several studies where women stopped all caffeine, the lumpiness to the breast remained unchanged. However, some women do report that they do have less breast pain.

Q. **Does taking Vitamin E help prevent fibrocystic breast changes?**

A. There is no conclusive scientific evidence that Vitamin E has any beneficial effect.

Q. **Do fibrocystic changes in my breast make me more likely to develop breast cancer?**

A. Probably 90 percent of the fibrocystic changes seen on breast biopsies have little effect on increasing a woman's risk of breast cancer. The only changes that significantly increase the chance of breast cancer are microscopic cellular changes called proliferative changes and atypia changes ***(See Chapter 7)***.

Q. **Does breast lumpiness vary among women?**

A. Yes. Lumpiness varies greatly with menstrual cycle fluctuations. It also varies according to the amount or ratio of the different breast tissues. Breasts that have more fibrous or dense connective tissue feel more lumpy. Women with more fat tissue covering the breast tissue have much softer and less lumpy breasts because the normal breast tissue is not felt as easily under the fat.

Q. **Are my lumpy breasts the result of a hormone imbalance?**

A. In the past, it was thought that an imbalance of estrogen, progesterone, and prolactin which stimulate growth of breast cells may contribute to abnormal lumpiness. Presently, there is no agreement on this subject. Measuring hormone levels is not helpful since the levels fluctuate dramatically throughout a normal menstrual cycle.

Q. **I have not had any children. Does that explain why my breasts are so hard and lumpy?**

A. Women who have never given birth sometimes have firmer, lumpier breasts in their thirties and forties, compared to women who have had children.

Q. **Does having firm, lumpy breasts increase my chance of developing breast cancer?**

A. Probably not. Only tissue changes that are associated with an increased risk are those called proliferative changes. This is a descriptive phrase used by pathologists describing the tissue changes seen only through a microscope. Fortunately, this tissue finding is uncommon and is not necessarily associated with lumpy breasts.

Chapter Five

BREAST PAIN and NIPPLE PROBLEMS

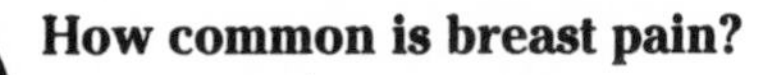

Q. **How common is breast pain?**

A. Breast pain (mastalgia), especially that which is premenstrual, is very common. Studies show 50 percent of women experience breast pain sometime.

Q. **Is breast pain related to breast cancer?**

A. Breast pain is an uncommon symptom of breast cancer, occurring only about 5 percent to 10 percent of the time, usually in the case of smaller tumors, most often lobular cancer. The pain is constant in position and is unrelated to the cyclical pain of menstrual cycles.

Q. **Are there different types of breast pain?**

A. Pain is pain; however, doctors divide breast pain into two types. The first and most common type is cyclical pain. It is premenstrual and may last as long as a week or more. Usually felt in both breasts, cyclical pain may be worse in the upper-outer quadrant of the breast and may be worse in one breast than in the other. The pain has been described as a heaviness and tenderness to the touch, and it can radiate to the armpit area or down the inner arm. It is often accompanied by nodularity or lumpiness in the breast.

The second type of breast pain is noncyclical and is unrelated to the menstrual cycle. It occurs in both pre- and postmenopausal women and usually affects only one breast. It is more likely to be in the inner quadrant of the breast or behind the nipple. Often described as burning, drawing, or tenderness to touch, the pain is made worse with cold. Nodularity or lumpiness in the breast is not present as often as in cases of cyclical pain.

Trauma from an injury, a previous abscess, or biopsy can also be the cause of noncyclical pain. Fortunately, pain from trauma will usually disappear with time. Other possible causes of noncyclical breast pain are duct ectasia, sclerosing adenosis, and fat necrosis ***(See Chapter 7 for definition)***.

With noncyclical pain, mammogram abnormalities such as coarse calcification, ductal dilatation, or fat necrosis are more likely to be seen.

Q. **A friend told me that after I started menopause my breast pain would stop. Is this true?**

A. Menopause, when there are lower levels of hormones present, does bring relief to the majority of women who suffer from breast pain. However, for women on hormone replacement therapy, the pain only lessens; it does not completely disappear.

Q. **Can pain originating in the breasts be felt in the upper inner arms?**

A. Yes. Major nerve trunks that go to the breasts also go to the armpit areas and the upper arms, creating the phenomenon called "referred pain." This is similar to what happens when a heart attack victim feels pain in the left arm. A pinched nerve in the neck can also cause pain in the breast if that nerve eventually goes to the breast.

Q. **Can rib problems cause breast pain?**

A. Yes. Pain originating from the place where the ribs join the cartilage of the sternum (breast bone) can cause pain. This rib pain is called Tietze's syndrome. It can occur at any age and is usually located on only one side of the chest. Anti-inflammatory drugs like aspirin generally relieve the discomfort.

Q. **Can increased fluid retention at the time of my period be causing my breast pain?**

A. Studies show that the amount of fluids retained by women who have breast pain is no different than that of women who do not have breast pain.

Q. **Some people have told me that my breast pain is the result of psychological problems. Is this true?**

A. Studies of personality traits of women who have and do not have breast pain have failed to show any psychological abnormality in women who complain of breast pain.

Q. **Are my painful breasts caused from a hormone irregularity?**

A. Studies show that there is no difference in the estrogen or progesterone levels in women who have painful nodular breasts compared to women who do not have these symptoms. What has been discovered recently is that women with painful breasts may have a disturbance in the pituitary gland, causing more prolactin to be secreted in an erratic fashion. Why the pituitary gland secretions are increased and erratic in women with painful breasts is a mystery.

Q. **Can taking birth control pills cause me to have breast pain?**

A. Breast pain is often experienced after a woman starts taking birth control pills; however, most of the pain disappears after she has taken them for several months. If the pain becomes severe, changing to a lower-dose estrogen pill or to a different brand of pills may be advisable. If breast pain continues to be a problem, it would be worthwhile to stop using oral contraceptives to determine if the pills were indeed the cause of the pain.

Q. **What drugs have been tried for severe breast pain that is cyclical in nature?**

A. **1.** Diuretics, or "water pills," have been tried but seem to have little beneficial effect.
2. Progesterone hormone therapy is presently being evaluated but cannot be recommended at this time.
3. Tamoxifen, an estrogen-blocking hormone, has been helpful in reducing cyclical breast pain; however, the FDA has approved its use for the treatment of breast cancer only. If it proves to be low in toxicity when used for the prevention of breast cancer, it may become available for the treatment of cyclical breast pain.
4. Bromocriptine decreases cyclical breast pain in approximately 50 percent of cases, but how it does it remains a mystery, and the FDA has not approved it for this use. It is, however, used after childbirth to prevent the formation of breast milk. It is also used to counteract the effect of too much prolactin from pituitary tumors and to treat Parkinson's disease.
5. Danazol, a synthetic testosterone, relieves cyclical breast pain in approximately 70 percent of women; however, it can lower a woman's voice and cause menstrual irregularity. Although it works well in relieving cyclical breast pain, the male side effects of the drug limit its use.
6. Evening primrose oil, a rich source of essential fatty acids, was first reported in 1981 as an aid in relieving cyclical breast pain. Available in most health food stores, the normal dosage is 300 mg per day, and there are no known side effects. About 50 percent of women report this treatment to be helpful; however, it takes about four to six weeks before any effect can be appreciated.
7. In the 1960s, Vitamin E was reported to relieve cyclical breast pain, although two double-blind studies reported in 1985 failed to demonstrate any beneficial effects. These

studies have not dissuaded some women from taking 400 units of Vitamin E a day, with the hope that it will provide some relief.

8. Caffeine was reported in 1979 as a cause of breast pain and nodularity, although two controlled, double-blind studies since then have failed to prove this. But because caffeine has been thought to be associated with many health problems in the past, stopping all consumption of caffeine is often recommended to see if its absence has any effect on the patient's breast pain.

9. Vitamins A and B_6 have been tried on small test groups of patients with cyclical breast pain, but the results are questionable.

10. Pregnancy and menopause generally bring relief of cyclical breast pain, although these conditions have little effect on noncyclical breast pain.

11. Fortunately, breast pain does have periods of natural remission. For this reason, it is often difficult to identify the reasons why breast pain comes and goes.

Q. **What drugs or treatment are available for noncyclical breast pain?**

A. **1.** Danazol, Bromocriptine, and evening primrose oil have all been shown to relieve noncyclical breast pain, but they are more effective for relief of cyclical breast pain.

2. If a woman has a persistent area that causes pain, the area can be injected with a local anesthetic mixed with a steroid. This injection treatment can be repeated several times.

3. The painful area of the breast can also be surgically removed. This treatment is considered if the area is painful to the touch and if the pain can be relieved by the use of local anesthetic injection. Approximately 50 percent of women can be helped by this procedure, but few women find the pain severe enough to choose surgery.

Q. **How often are biopsies done for nipple discharge?**

A. In one study of 1,253 patients having breast biopsies, nipple discharge was the symptom in only 8 percent of all the breast biopsies.

Q. **Is it normal for a woman to have any nipple discharge?**

A. Fluid is contained naturally in the milk ducts, and it is not uncommon to be able to express a few drops of gray or green discharge from the nipple with firm squeezing. When the nipple is squeezed or stimulated, nervous impulses travel from the breast to the brain, commanding the pituitary gland to release prolactin, a hormone that stimulates the breast to make milk. Consequently, when the breast or nipple is squeezed repeatedly, secretions may begin to occur. One study reports that fluid could be expressed in 83 percent of breast examinations.

Q. **Is nipple discharge always the same?**

A. There are several different types of nipple discharge: milky, sticky and multi-colored pus, clear or watery, yellow, pink, and bloody.

Q. **What type of discharge is most likely to indicate cancer?**

A. If the discharge is from one breast only, and from a single duct, it is more apt to be cancer, especially if there is blood in the discharge. The discharge should also be persistent and spontaneous, not related to breast-feeding.

Q. **How often does nipple discharge occur in women with cancer?**

A. Nipple discharge probably occurs in about one percent to five percent of patients with breast cancer. In most of these cases, the women have a lump or an abnormality that showed up on a mammogram.

Q. **How often does nipple discharge indicate cancer?**

A. A 1989 study reports the following:

Type of discharge	Percent Cancer
Clear yellow	6%
Blood-tinged	13%
Bloody	27%
Watery	33%

Q. **Is it beneficial to evaluate the discharge fluid from the nipple?**

A. A large number of false negative reports have made this matter the subject of debate. My feeling is that examination of the fluid is only helpful if the report is positive for cancer.

Q. **Can a pregnancy cause bloody nipple discharge?**

A. During the second or third trimester of the first or second pregnancy, a small blood-stained nipple discharge can occur occasionally.

Q. **I had galactorrhea. What is that?**

A. Galactorrhea is the secretion of a milky-like fluid from the breasts during periods when the breasts should not be making milk.

Although approximately one-third of the cases result from unknown causes, galactorrhea often occurs with amenorrhea (absence of menstrual period) or ovulatory dysfunction. Some cases result from increased prolactin or progesterone levels; however, in approximately one-third of the cases there is either no elevation in the level of prolactin or a cause for the increased prolactin can not be found.

Galactorrhea can also be caused by medications, particularly those drugs which cause the pituitary gland to produce inappropriate secretions of prolactin. Some of the drugs that might cause galactorrhea include Thyroxine, Aldomet (used to treat hypertension), estrogen, progesterone, and H_2 blockers such as Cimetidine (Tagamet).

Hyperthyroidism and thyroid insufficiency, chest wall trauma, mastectomy, herpes infections, or shingles of the chest wall have also been found to increase prolactin secretion and galactorrhea.

When persistent galactorrhea occurs, especially with elevated prolactin, a physician may order a CAT scan of the brain to determine if there is a pituitary gland tumor. If there is no evidence of a tumor and all other causes of inappropriate prolactin secretion are discounted, careful follow-up and monitoring of the problem is all that is needed. If a woman has severe galactorrhea and no cause for it can be found, she may be treated with drugs that will counteract the prolactin and relieve her symptoms.

Chapter Six

PREGNANCY CHANGES AND BREAST-FEEDING

Q. What percentage of mothers breast-feed their children?

A. We don't know exactly how many, but we do know the percentage of women breast-feeding is increasing. In 1970, approximately 25 percent of women giving birth were breast-feeding the baby at one week of age, but by 1985 this figure had increased to 60 percent. The incidence of breast-feeding begins to decrease among mothers of infants five months of age. In 1970, the figure was approximately 5 percent; by 1984, the percentage had only increased to 27 percent.

Studies indicate that women who elect to breast-feed their infants are generally more educated, more mature, and enjoy a higher economical lifestyle than those who do not breast-feed.

Q. **When a breast is squeezed, is a nipple discharge normal?**

A. Some nipple discharge is normal. The ducts of the breast are filled with fluid and cells, so when the nipples are squeezed, the ducts are irritated and a small amount of these cells and fluid are discharged. Also, when the nipple is squeezed or stimulated, nervous impulses are sent from the breast to the brain, causing the pituitary gland to release prolactin, the hormone that stimulates the breast to make milk.

Q. **How prevalent is breast cancer among pregnant women?**

A. Approximately 3 percent of all breast cancers occur in pregnant women.

Q. **What is the average age of pregnant women who develop breast cancer?**

A. Breast cancer usually occurs in the older pregnant woman, and the average age is approximately 32 to 35 years of age.

Q. **Is breast cancer worse if one is pregnant?**

A. This is often true because when breast cancer is diagnosed during a pregnancy, it is generally diagnosed late and the cancer is in a more advanced stage. This delay in diagnosis occurs because the breast, during pregnancy, is difficult to examine. During pregnancy, the breast undergoes many changes, making it difficult to determine which changes are abnormal and which are normal. Also, mammography has difficulty detecting cancer in a pregnant breast.

In addition, many women who are pregnant are very reluctant to undergo a breast biopsy because they are afraid it will harm their developing child.

Many physicians believe that the delay in diagnosis makes breast cancer in a pregnant woman seem more aggressive than it really is.

Q. **Does breast cancer have any effect on a woman's pregnancy?**

A. Only the treatment of the cancer—surgery, chemotherapy, or radiation—affects a pregnancy.

Q. **Are there any benign conditions of the breast that can become worse with pregnancy or breast-feeding?**

A. In general, benign conditions of the breast do not cause any problems with the breast once it begins lactation during pregnancy. Sometimes, however, lactation can trigger problems if the woman has large fibroadenomas ***(see Chapter 7)***. Also, fibroadenomas can sometimes grow quickly during pregnancy, causing a painful, hard mass in the breast.

Q. **If a breast cancer develops or is discovered during pregnancy, should it be treated immediately, or should the woman wait until after the baby is delivered?**

A. Treatment of breast cancer should begin immediately, even though the woman is pregnant. Delayed treatment might result in a minimal disease becoming an advanced disease.

Q. **If a pregnant patient develops breast cancer, is the treatment any different than that for a non-pregnant patient?**

A. The difference is only in the consideration of radiation therapy. Because the long-term effects of radiation on a developing baby—even in minute doses—are not known, most physicians favor a total mastectomy.

Q. **If a pregnant woman develops breast cancer, can she still receive adjuvant chemotherapy after her surgery?**

A. Yes. Adjuvant chemotherapy has been given to pregnant women in the first, second, and third trimesters. However, different chemotherapy agents have more toxicity, and the long term effects on children exposed to these agents is not known, nor do we know the exact incidence of malformations resulting from chemotherapy.

All chemotherapy agents increase the risk of damage to the developing child, and since every type of chemotherapeutic agent has different risks, it is important to fully discuss the advantages and disadvantages of any chemotherapy with the treating oncologist.

Q. **Once a woman has been treated for breast cancer, can she safely become pregnant again?**

A. Studies report that getting pregnant again is safe, as long as there is no evidence of metastasis or cancer spread when the pregnancy begins. Because cancer grows much more quickly during pregnancy, it is important for the woman who has had cancer to be certain she is cancer-free before getting pregnant again. Most physicians recommend waiting at least two to five years after the initial treatment before trying to conceive again.

Q. **When a woman is pregnant and discovers she has breast cancer, are the survival risks higher or lower?**

A. Not many studies have been completed in this area, but the few conducted revealed the survival of pregnant and non-pregnant women did not differ if the women were matched for age and stage at diagnosis.

Q. **If I eat a low-fat, low-cholesterol diet while breast-feeding, will the milk I manufacture have less fat? And will my milk be better for my child?**

A. Not necessarily. The concentration of fats in human milk is very uniform and does not deviate very much, nor does your diet greatly affect its consistency. The amount of cholesterol in milk is approximately 20 milligrams per three ounces and will not change with dietary manipulation.

Q. **I've read that a woman's milk is more easily digested than either formula or cow's milk. Is this true?**

A. Yes. Breast milk is digested twice as fast as formula milk (two hours for breast milk as compared to four hours for formula).

Q. **How does breast-feeding benefit my baby?**

A. One of the most important benefits of breast-feeding is that it provides the infant protection against bacteria and viruses. The milk that a mother first produces has a high amount of IgA, an immunoglobulin which helps protect the baby from viruses and bacterial toxins. IgA also protects the baby from developing allergies later in life. After the baby reaches two to three months of age, it is able to make its own IgA immunoglobulin, but until then, the mother's milk is its only source. Additional immunoglobulins, as well as other ingredients that increase the baby's resistance to infections, are also contained in breast milk.

Another benefit of breast-feeding is that babies are able to digest breast milk much more quickly than formula and have much less diarrhea.

Q. **At what point in the pregnancy are breasts ready to produce milk?**

A. The breasts have grown and are ready to start producing milk by approximately 20 weeks of pregnancy; however, large amounts of progesterone in the blood stream prevent them from manufacturing milk at this time. Once the baby is born and the progesterone level decreases, increased levels of the hormones prolactin and oxytocin cause the breasts to start making milk.

Q. **Explain how a mother's milk comes (lets down) when her baby sucks, or when she simply hears its cry.**

A. When the mother hears her baby's cry, the hypothalamus gland (located in the brain) releases oxytocin, which causes the muscle cells in the breast to squeeze the glandular and ductal tissue. This causes the milk to be ejected from the nipple.

When the baby sucks on the mother's nipple, this stimulates nerve receptors in the area which also cause the release of oxytocin. Increased levels of the hormone prolactin are also released into the bloodstream when the baby sucks. This hormone, also secreted by the hypothalamus, is the main hormone which stimulates the breast cells to manufacture milk.

Q. **What is necessary to ensure that my breasts will continue to produce milk?**

A. Stimulation of the nipple and areola (dark area surrounding the nipple) and the removal of the milk from the breast are the most important factors. If the infant fails to suck properly, the hypothalamus (a special gland in the brain) will not release prolactin in large enough levels to continue to tell the breasts to make milk. The nipples and areola *must* be stimulated for milk production to continue.

Q. **Will breast augmentation (implants) or breast reduction surgery interfere with my ability to breast-feed?**

A. Breast augmentation is unlikely to interfere with breast-feeding because the implant is placed behind the breast tissue. Breast reduction surgery, however, *can* interfere because the nerves going to the nipples may be damaged. Also, the ducts draining the breasts may be damaged or develop scar tissue around them so that milk can not get out of the breast through the ducts.

Q. **If I have small breasts, will I be unable to breast-feed?**

A. A small-breasted woman seldom has any problem breast-feeding. The glandular tissue in her breasts will increase in volume and, with proper stimulation, will manufacture enough milk to breast-feed successfully.

Q. **If I intend to breast-feed, how soon after my baby's birth can I begin?**

A. The best time to start breast-feeding is as soon after birth as possible—within one hour. At this time, the milk available for the baby is called colostrum and is richer in proteins and antibodies than the milk which is produced later.

Q. How often should I feed my newborn baby?

A. A newborn will probably want to be fed every two to three hours, requiring approximately eight to ten feedings in a 24-hour period.

Q. When I start breast-feeding, should I feed from only one breast at each feeding, or from both breasts?

A. In the beginning, it is probably best to use both breasts at each breast-feeding, starting with the breast nursed from last. Later, after your milk has been established and you have determined which breast satisfies the baby most, it is possible to feed the baby from only one breast at a time at each feeding. It is important, however, to use both breasts equally during the months of breast-feeding to avoid causing one breast to become larger than the other.

Q. Do I have to take any special care of my nipples when breast-feeding?

A. The nipples have special oil glands on them called Montgomery's glands that lubricate the nipples with natural oils. For this reason, the nipples should not be washed with soap, but they should be cleansed with water to remove any milk residue. This should be enough to keep the nipples clean and to prevent them from developing any cracks.

Q. I have inverted nipples. Will I be able to breast-feed?

A. Most women with inverted nipples are able to breast-feed by placing special shells on the nipples to make them overt (protrude). These may be worn in the last trimester of pregnancy. Also, exercises called Hoffmans can be done after delivery to help make the nipple overt more easily.

Q. **A friend of mine had an infection in her breasts while breast-feeding. Is this very common?**

A. Fortunately, infection of breasts (mastitis) is not very common. In some cases, surgery may be required to drain the abscess, but most of the time it can be cured with antibiotics and local heat.

Q. **If I do not want to breast-feed, are there drugs which my doctor can give me to prevent me from making milk after I have delivered?**

A. Yes, there are several drugs, especially Parlodel, which can be given to stop the manufacture of milk, but they are seldom necessary. If a woman wears a well-fitting bra and does not stimulate her breasts, she will probably not need any drugs to prevent her from making milk. If her milk does come in and her breasts become engorged, taking warm showers and applying cool compresses will relieve discomfort while waiting for her breasts to stop making milk.

Q. **Can breast-feeding spread AIDS?**

A. The virus causing human immunodeficiency virus (HIV) has been found in the milk of women who are HIV positive. For this reason, it is probably not wise for a woman who has tested positive for human immunodeficiency virus to breast-feed a baby. If the baby tests positive for AIDS at birth, breast-feeding by the mother probably makes no difference.

Q. **What is a galactocele?**

A. A galactocele is a breast cyst that is filled with milk. It can become a palpable mass, much like a lump or other abnormality, and for that reason a woman may become alarmed by its discovery. But a galactocele can be aspirated to prevent infection and to reassure the woman that she has not developed a lump that is suspicious for cancer.

Q. **If I have breast cancer in a breast, would that breast continue to make milk and will the baby take the milk?**

A. The breast with breast cancer will continue to make milk until the cancer becomes so large there are no normal cells to make milk.

It has been suggested that a nursing infant may reject the milk from a cancerous breast, but this has never been proven.

Q. **If I drink alcohol, will the alcohol go into my breast milk?**

A. Yes, alcohol does go into the breast milk within 30 minutes after consumption, and the effects of alcohol on the baby are directly related to the amount the mother ingests.

Q. **Does smoking affect breast-feeding?**

A. Yes. Cigarette smoking usually complicates breast-feeding. The nicotine from the cigarettes goes into the breast milk and may very well affect the baby's health and behavior.

Q. **Does caffeine go into breast milk?**

A. Yes, caffeine does go into the breast milk, but it probably does not significantly stimulate the baby unless the woman drinks approximately five or more cups of coffee or caffeine beverages a day.

Q. **Do most of the drugs I take go into breast milk?**

A. Yes, most drugs that are consumed go into breast milk in varying concentrations. If you have to take any drugs while breast-feeding, it is very important for you to discuss this with your baby's pediatrician and the physician ordering the drug to see if it will have any effect on your baby.

Q. **How important is diet while breast-feeding?**

A. Diet is very important, because the breasts utilize or steal all of the necessary nutrients to make its high-quality milk. If the mother does not have the necessary nutrients, she will be affected, along with the milk she produces.

Q. **I have heard that it is possible to lose weight while breast-feeding. Is this true?**

A. A nursing mother will burn approximately 500 calories more per day than a non-nursing mother. This is because calories are used in the manufacture of the milk, and additional calories are fed to the child when the milk is consumed. For this reason nursing mothers will often lose more weight than non-nursing mothers.

Q. **Does breast-feeding prevent me from becoming pregnant?**

A. Although breast-feeding is known to retard ovulation, after three months it has very little effect on decreasing the possibility of pregnancy. Overall, using breast-feeding to decrease the possibility of pregnancy is not a very wise decision, because it is not very reliable.

Q. **I have felt sexually aroused with the baby sucking on my nipples. Is this normal?**

A. It is normal for some women to feel sexual arousal because the elevation of prolactin affects the pelvic organs. It is also possible for a woman's breasts to release milk during sex.

Q. **If I eat a low-cholesterol diet, will I be able to decrease the amount of cholesterol in my milk?**

A. No. The amount of cholesterol in breast milk is stable, regardless of the levels in your diet.

Q. **How good are the breast pumps which are available to express milk if I am not able to breast-feed on schedule?**

A. Some mechanical pump devices are very good, but they must be used frequently, according to your normal breast-feeding schedule, to ensure that your breasts are stimulated enough to continue producing milk. Since there are a variety of breast pumps available, you may want to ask a lactation consultant for the most current information.

Q. **How long will breast milk be adequate nutrition for the baby?**

A. Breast milk gives a baby complete nutrition for approximately four to six months.

Q. **If I am going to stop breast-feeding, is it better to stop slowly or to stop all at once?**

A. Gradual weaning will be best for both baby and mother. Eliminating one daily feeding no more often than every two or three days allows the mother's milk supply to decrease slowly without fullness or discomfort. If a woman abruptly stops breast-feeding, she is likely to experience painful engorgement of the breasts and can develop plugged ducts or mastitis. If a woman has to stop breast-feeding abruptly, taking aspirin, wearing a well-fitting bra, applying ice packs to the breast, and taking warm showers will relieve any discomfort and will help stop the natural leaking of milk as production stops naturally.

A note of caution: Binding the breasts is an outdated practice than can intensify a mother's discomfort and cause plugged ducts.

Q. **Is it normal for my nipples to become more erect during pregnancy and to become darker in color?**

A. Yes. Under the influence of increased hormones during pregnancy, the breasts are stimulated so that the nipple becomes more pigmented and more erect. The nipple never completely loses the pigmentation once the mother has delivered the baby.

Q. **My breasts became very warm during my last pregnancy. Is this normal?**

A. When the breast is undergoing the changes of pregnancy, there is increased blood flow because of the rapid growth of breast tissue. Also, the blood vessels are dilated (enlarged).

Q. **If I develop a breast infection (mastitis) while breast-feeding, will it be necessary for me to stop nursing my baby?**

A. No. Mastitis does *not* require you to stop breast-feeding. In fact, the best treatment for a quick recovery is to continue to breast-feed. Applying moist heat to the breast, increasing fluid intake, bed rest, and the cautious use of antibiotics will also aid in healing a breast infection.

Chapter Seven

BREAST BIOPSIES AND TISSUE RESULTS

Q&A **What are the different types of breast biopsies?**

There are two types. The first type is called an incisional biopsy in which only a portion of the lump or abnormality is removed. The second type is called an excisional biopsy where the entire lump or abnormality is removed. Some women refer to this type of biopsy as a lumpectomy.

Q. **What are the different ways to do a biopsy?**

A. There are three ways. The first technique, which gives the smallest sample, is a cytological preparation, called a fine-needle aspiration, or FNA. The second type is a core biopsy which yields a sample the size of a pencil lead. The last type is an open biopsy in which the entire lump or a portion of it is removed using a surgical excision.

Q. **How is a fine-needle aspiration (FNA) performed?**

A. When a fine-needle biopsy is performed, a needle the size that is used to give a patient a regular injection is pushed in and out of a palpable lump, withdrawing a small number of cells for analysis. The procedure is performed in a physician's office and is not very painful. Local anesthesia is not always necessary.

Q. **What are the advantages and disadvantages of fine-needle aspiration to determine the type of tissue in a palpable breast lump?**

A. The advantages are that it is safe, simple, inexpensive, and fast. The disadvantage is that its accuracy rate can be from 75 percent to 95 percent. If the FNA is performed by an experienced physician, the accuracy rate is closer to 95 percent; however, in the best of hands a small number of missed cancers cannot be avoided. Since FNA is not 100 percent accurate, one needs to use the information gained from physical exams and mammography to help determine if any other treatment is needed for a palpable breast lump. FNA has been used by some physicians for nonpalpable breast masses seen on mammography, but its acceptance is controversial for lesions seen only on mammography.

Q. **What is a core biopsy?**

A. When a core biopsy is performed, a special needle is used to remove a sample of tissue about the diameter of a fine pencil lead and about one-half-inch long. The needle requires a skin incision about one-eighth inch long, so local anesthesia is used. Core biopsies are performed in a physician's office or in an X-ray suite if the procedure is sampling tissue from an abnormality seen on mammography or ultrasound.

A core biopsy yields a larger tissue sample than does FNA. This is important to pathologists who will be evaluating the findings, because the more tissue they have to evaluate, the more accurate they can be.

Q. **What are the advantages and disadvantages of a core biopsy?**

A. A core biopsy, like a fine-needle aspiration, is safe, simple, relatively inexpensive, and doesn't take long to perform. Most patients who are candidates for surgical biopsy can also be evaluated with a core biopsy. Core biopsies can also be used for nonpalpable lesions, because the needle can be directed either sonographically or using mammography. The disadvantages of core biopsies are that they can, of course, miss the lesion; or they may sample only a portion of the lesion—perhaps that portion which does not show a malignancy, and the findings can then be misleading.

Most doctors feel core biopsies are not appropriate for calcifications seen on mammograms because they can miss a cancer that might be nearby. Having said all this, the accuracy for a core biopsy probably approaches 90 percent. However, as with a fine-needle aspiration, the core biopsy cannot remove the palpable mass or abnormality that the mammogram revealed. Core biopsy procedures must be followed with close physical exams and mammography to make sure the lesion is stable. If the lesion appears to grow or change, a repeat core biopsy or an open biopsy would be necessary.

Q. **What is an open-breast biopsy?**

A. When an open-breast biopsy is performed, the breast is "opened," an incision made so that the abnormality (either all or a portion of it) which had been palpated or viewed by mammography can be removed. Anesthesia may be either general or local, and the procedure is generally performed in an operating room. The main disadvantages of an open-breast biopsy are the costs, the surgical scar and the anxiety that people experience going into an operating room. Fortunately, most breast biopsies can be performed in ambulatory surgery centers where the costs are considerably less than those incurred in a hospital operating room. Also, the experience in an ambulatory surgery is less frightening because most patients coming into that setting are much healthier and the surrounding equipment is less intimidating.

Q. **What is a wire localization?**

A. A wire localization is performed on a woman who has an

abnormality in the breast that can only be seen by mammography or sonograpahy and cannot be felt. In such cases, about an hour prior to surgery, the woman is sent to radiology for a mammogram. The radiologist immediately reads the film, locates the lesion or abnormality, and then calculates the direction for inserting a wire into the breast toward the lesion. Once the wire is inserted, another mammogram is performed, making sure the wire has indeed reached the abnormality. Next, with the wire in place, the patient goes to the operating room, and a surgeon then uses the wire as a guide, following it to the lesion that needs to be removed. The surgeon removes the wire, taking with it tissue that will be sent to the radiologist to be compared with the size and shape of the abnormality seen on the mammogram. The tissue will then be evaluated by a pathologist.

Wire localization may seem like a complicated procedure, but remember: it is used to locate a lump or lesion that is only seen by mammography or sonography. The use of the wire and the additional mammograms enable the surgeon to locate and reach the abnormality without having to cut away a large amount of normal breast.

Q. **Approximately what percentage of breast biopsies turn out to be malignant?**

A. Of open-breast biopsies performed in the United States, approximately 25 percent turn out to be malignant. Of fine-needle aspirations and core biopsies, the chance of malignancy is probably much less since these techniques are most often used in instances where the likelihood of malignancy is much lower.

Q. **What type of surgeons treat breast diseases and perform breast surgery?**

A. General surgeons perform most of the breast cancer surgery and treatment of the benign breast problems in the

United States. It is unusual for plastic surgeons to treat breast cancer; they generally restrict their territory to the reconstruction of the breasts after the cancer has been removed.

Q. **What kind of training is required for a general surgeon?**

A. After they complete medical school, general surgeons spend at least five years in general surgical training. They are trained in the treatment of surgical disorders of the breasts, abdomen, endocrine glands, vascular system, orthopedic fractures, soft-tissue problems, and thoracic and traumatic surgery.

Q. **Is it better to go to a breast surgeon or a general surgeon?**

A. Breast surgeons are usually general surgeons who have restricted their practice to the surgical treatment of breast disorders. Breast surgery is not considered especially difficult, so surgeons who restrict themselves to breast surgery *only* may lose some of their "edge" when it comes to more complicated kinds of surgery. My opinion is that patients are best served if they see general surgeons whose treatment of breast disorders represents at least one-third of their total practice. Obviously, a very important factor is the patient's peace of mind. She should find a surgeon she feels comfortable with and one who can answer her questions in an understandable manner so that she can make informed and intelligent decisions regarding treatment.

Q. **How dangerous is a breast biopsy and what are the complications?**

A. A breast biopsy has minimal risks. In a fine-needle aspiration or a core biopsy, the main complications are bleeding and infection. Both of these complications occur only about 1 percent to 2 percent of the time and are usually easily corrected. An open breast biopsy performed in an operating room can also be complicated by bleeding and infection, but again, these occur only 1 percent to 2 percent of the time. Local or general anesthesia, which is administered for an open biopsy, adds the only other risk associated with this procedure.

Q. **What should I do if I've felt a lump in my breast? Do all lumps need to be biopsied?**

A. The first thing one should do is see a physician who is skilled in palpating lumps. If he or she feels the lump is not really a lump, possibly nothing will need to be done. Because breasts change with the menstrual cycle, sometimes a doctor will recommend waiting a cycle to see if, as often happens, the lump changes or goes away.

The next step is to have a mammogram, even if the patient is in her thirties. This will help determine if an abnormality requiring a biopsy is present in the breast. If no abnormality is seen on the mammogram, the physician may want to try to aspirate the mass to see if it is solid or cystic. (It should be emphasized that a normal mammogram does not ensure that cancer is not present.) If the mass is a simple cyst, aspiration draws the fluid out and the lump will disappear.

If the cyst recurs three times, the surgeon may want to remove it to prevent its persistent recurring. If the mass is solid and does not disappear by placing a needle in it, then the surgeon may want to biopsy it, using one of the procedures explained above—fine-needle aspiration, core, or open biopsy. If a fine-needle aspiration or core biopsy is performed and shows the mass to be benign, the surgeon will probably want to follow this mass, examining it again at regular intervals to make sure it is not changing or growing. If an open breast biopsy is performed and the entire mass is removed, the patient is relieved of the worrisome presence of a lump in the breast and the concern about its possible recurrence.

Q. **You stated that approximately 25 percent of all open-breast biopsies in the U.S. reveal the presence of cancer. Do I have to wait until the chance of cancer is that high before I have an open-breast biopsy?**

A. No. Some women want to undergo an open-breast biopsy even if the chance of the mass being malignant is only 1 percent. Surgeons always prefer to do an open-breast biopsy if they feel there is a malignancy, or if they feel it will greatly relieve the patient's mind. I believe it is important for women to know the chances of malignancy, and then the decision to undergo an open-breast biopsy should be theirs. For many women, the peace of mind they gain by learning they do not have breast cancer far outweighs the discomforts associated with an open-breast biopsy.

Q. **I understand I can find out the results of my breast biopsy right away if a frozen section is performed. What is a frozen section?**

A. A frozen section is a procedure performed on the breast tissue by a pathologist. The pathologist processes the tissue quickly by freezing it, cutting it into thin sections, and then applying special stains. The process takes only about 5–10 minutes. Frozen sections are not always necessary for a diagnosis and, at some hospitals, the cost for this procedure can be almost as much as the surgical fee.

Q. **What criteria are used in deciding to do a frozen section?**

A. Before a frozen section can be performed, there must be enough tissue removed to be able to make a correct diagnosis by both frozen and permanent tissue-processing techniques. In most cases, the available tissue for examination must be larger than three-eighth's inch before the pathologist will perform a frozen section. The pathologist always wants to have enough tissue left over to do permanent tissue processing, which takes 24 hours. This is the only way a definitive diagnosis is made.

Q. **Why would a pathologist be reluctant to perform a frozen section on tissue removed from a breast?**

A. Pathologists never want to do a frozen section if they feel there is any chance the diagnosis could be compromised. In detecting subtle atypical ductal changes or microinvasion, frozen sections are not reliable. Some cancer and malignant papillary lesions are also very difficult to diagnose by frozen section. Also, fatty tissue, of which the breast is composed, cannot be frozen and cut effectively, hindering the pathologist from accurately determining the margins around the tumor. In cases where there is no gross lesion visible on the tissue removed, the pathologist will cut the tissue into many tiny slices and evaluate each portion. This procedure cannot be performed with a frozen section.

Microcalcification in a breast specimen without a visible mass often makes it challenging for the pathologist to determine if there is a small cancer present. Therefore, the pathologist will perform as many step sections (small slices) of the tissue as possible, looking for suspicious cells and calcifications. Multiple step sections can only be performed with permanent tissue processing.

Generally, if a woman has an available mass greater than one-half inch, a pathologist is able to conduct a frozen section and reach a diagnosis 80 percent to 90 percent of the time. If there is any question concerning the tissue removed, the pathologist will always defer a frozen section diagnosis and wait 24 to 48 hours to process the tissue in such a manner as to reach a more definitive diagnosis. Pathologists will often get a second opinion on the tissue if there is any question concerning malignancy.

Q. **What does the pathologist do with the tissue removed from the breast in the operating room?**

A. The tissue may be X-rayed if either the surgeon or pathologist feels the necessity to confirm that any suspicious area seen on the mammogram is in the tissue removed. The pathologist will also want to examine the tissue closely and measure both the size of the tissue and the abnormal tissue removed. The margins of the tissue removed will also be marked with ink and measured to determine the distance of any abnormal tissue from the margins of the specimen. A frozen section will be performed if the pathologist feels the final diagnosis will not be compromised. Hormone (estrogen and progesterone) receptors will also be evaluated to determine if the cancer is sensitive to hormones. Flow cytometry and various tissue growth factors may also be used to help determine the aggressiveness of the tumor cells. ***(See Chapter 8)***

Q. **The surgeon said that my breast biopsy showed that I had fibrocystic disease. What does that mean?**

A. The term "fibrocystic disease" is a misnomer, since the condition is not really a disease. But the term is in wide use by physicians, and it describes the normal aging process of the breasts. When a woman reaches the age of thirty, the glandular structure of her breasts starts to decrease and continues to decrease until she reaches her sixties or seventies. This is a normal process associated with aging; it is not a disease. Since all aspects of our bodies change as we grow older, it should be no surprise to us that the breast also undergoes changes with age.

Here is what happens as the breast ages. The connective tissue converts into dense collagen tissue (like sinew or tendon), giving the breast a more fibrous nature. Then later, the glandular structure and ducts start to die off (atrophy) and disappear. As they atrophy and disappear, cysts are sometimes formed as ducts are obstructed by the connective tissue or by the presence of extra cells in the ducts.

The tissue in the ducts may also show signs of aging by developing two or more layers of cells in the ducts, instead of the normal one to two layers of cells. When this change occurs, the condition is called hyperplasia, or proliferative changes.

As a woman becomes older, one of two things may occur: either the breasts become smaller as the breast tissue and connective tissue between the breast tissue decrease; or else the breasts become larger as fat replaces breast tissue.

Different areas of the breast age at different rates, causing some of the lumpiness women may feel in their breasts. As a woman continues to age and the entire breast is replaced by more fat, the lumpiness will diminish.

Q. **What is a fibroadenoma?**

A. A fibroadenoma is a benign tumor most commonly found in young women in their twenties and thirties. It can grow to be approximately one to two inches in size. Usually firm and smooth, a fibroadenoma probably occurs by the growth of connective tissue in the lobules. While most of these benign tumors are found in younger women, sometimes they may be detected in older women as well. When this happens it is generally believed that the tumors have been there since the woman's youth.

In approximately 80 percent to 90 percent of cases, only one fibroadenoma will be present in the breast; however, if a woman does develop one, she has approximately a 10–20 percent chance of developing a second tumor.

Fibroadenomas can grow quite quickly when they are stimulated by the increased hormones of pregnancy or oral contraceptives and, with age, they may harden and change into calcium.

Although some studies (New England Journal of Medicine, July 1994) have demonstrated a relationship between fibroadenomas and one's risk of developing breast cancer, it is not mandatory to remove a fibroadenoma if there is tissue confirmation that the mass is, in fact, a fibroadenoma. However, many patients want to have the fibroadenomas removed because they do not like the idea of living with a palpable mass in their breasts. Most surgeons will agree to remove these benign tumors to relieve both themselves and their patients of any palpable tumor masses.

In the future, with changes in the healthcare delivery system and concerns about economics, a simple needle biopsy may be all that is done to these abnormalities.

Q. **What is a papilloma?**

A. A papilloma could be compared to a mole occurring in the ducts of the breast. It is usually only a few millimeters in size and grows into the inside of the ducts. It can cause a bloody discharge from the nipple.

Papillomas should be removed. They are malignant approximately 5 percent of the time.

Q. **My pathology report says that I have duct ectasia. What is it?**

A. Duct ectasia is simply a normal aging process of the breasts in which the ducts leading to the nipple area dilate or become enlarged. It can cause some pain and nipple discharge. If secretions from the breast stagnate in the ducts, bacteria can grow in this fluid and cause the ducts to become infected. While the condition may be uncomfortable, duct ectasia is not serious and does not increase a woman's chance of developing breast cancer.

Q. **What is adenosis or sclerosing adenosis?**

A. Sclerosing adenosis describes a change of the breasts associated with aging. It occurs when the ductal tissue of the breast are packed extremely close together. Most physicians feel that sclerosing adenosis slightly increases one's risk of developing breast cancer.

Q. **My doctor said that I had fat necrosis from an old injury to my breast. What is fat necrosis?**

A. The term "fat necrosis" applies when the fat tissues of the breast have been injured, usually by trauma. The injury causes fat from the fat cells to leak out into the tissues, causing a chemical reaction. The result is an inflammation and a mass in the breast. Fat necrosis can also occur from radiation therapy for breast cancer and from the rupture of a cyst or a dilated duct in the breast tissue.

Fat necrosis is often mistaken for a cancer by mammography.

Q. **My doctor advised me I had intraductal hyperplasia on my breast biopsy report. What does that mean?**

A. Hyperplasia means the ducts which carry the milk from the lobules (lobules contain the acini which make the milk) to the nipple have developed an increased number of cells. Usually, one or two cells make up the walls in normal ducts, but when hyperplasia exists there is a thicker wall made up of more cells. A report of moderate to severe (florid) hyperplasia reflects an increase in the relative risk of breast cancer of about 1.5 to 2.0.

Q. **My pathology report shows that I have atypical hyperplasia. Is that worse than regular intraductal hyperplasia?**

A. Atypical hyperplasia means that the cells inside the duct do not appear completely normal. With atypical hyperplasia, the relative risk for breast cancer is increased to approximately 4. If a woman has a very strong positive family history of breast cancer, the chance is increased even more. Having atypical hyperplasia in one breast means that the chance of developing breast cancer is increased for either breast.

Q. **If I have intraductal hyperplasia with atypia, does that mean that I am always at increased risk for breast cancer?**

A. It is possible that this relative increased risk does not last for a lifetime; that as the breast ages and the duct cells are lost, a woman's chance of developing breast cancer may move toward the more normal relative risk of developing breast cancer. Some studies support the belief that a *premenopausal* woman is not always at risk of increased breast cancer if she has a biopsy showing hyperplasia or hyperplasia with atypia, but this is not known for sure and is controversial.

Of all breast biopsies performed, probably less than 15 percent show intraductal hyperplasia, and even less show intraductal hyperplasia with atypia.

Q. **What is ductal carcinoma in situ?**

A. Ductal carcinoma in situ means that the cells inside a duct have become malignant, but they have not left the duct, i.e., become invasive. Ductal carcinoma in situ means that the breast that has the ductal carcinoma in situ has a risk of developing invasive cancer. The exact increased risk is not completely known, because autopsy studies have shown many women to have ductal carcinoma in situ who never developed a known breast cancer during their lifetime. The incidence of ductal carcinoma in situ is increasing because it is being detected on mammography. It now comprises almost half of all cancer detected by mammography. For this reason, ductal carcinoma in situ may be a normal variant of a woman's breast, but this is very controversial. As the breast tissue ages, it is *possible* that many of this ductal carcinoma in situ regresses so that the increased risk factors do not persist for a woman's lifetime. (This is an optimistic theory and it is considered controversial.) Overall, if one has ductal carcinoma in situ, the increase in relative risk for developing invasive breast cancer is approximately 11, meaning that probably 25 percent of women who have ductal carcinoma in situ found by biopsy will go on to develop invasive breast cancer. ***(See drawing of cancer cells in situ, p. 84)***

Q. **Does ductal carcinoma in situ ever spread to the lymph nodes?**

A. It is quite unusual for ductal carcinoma to spread to the lymph nodes because the tumor has not left the ducts. Unless the tumor is very large, at least several inches in size, the chance of the cancer spreading to the axillary lymph nodes would be 0 percent to 1 percent.

Q. **Are there different types of ductal carcinoma in situ?**

A. Yes. Ductal carcinoma has been broken down into two groups: high grade and low grade. The high grade intraductal carcinoma in situ has a much higher chance of developing into invasive breast cancer than does the low grade.

The main type of high grade ductal carcinoma in situ is called "comedo." Doctors can identify this tumor by the presence of dead cells within the tumor and by the abnormal appearance of the cells and their very rapid division rate. A woman who has a high grade ductal cell carcinoma has a much better chance of developing recurrent cancer in her breasts no matter what type of treatment she receives, either local excision with no radiation or excision with radiation. The high grade ductal carcinoma has a greater chance of having spread to the axillary lymph nodes than does the low grade.

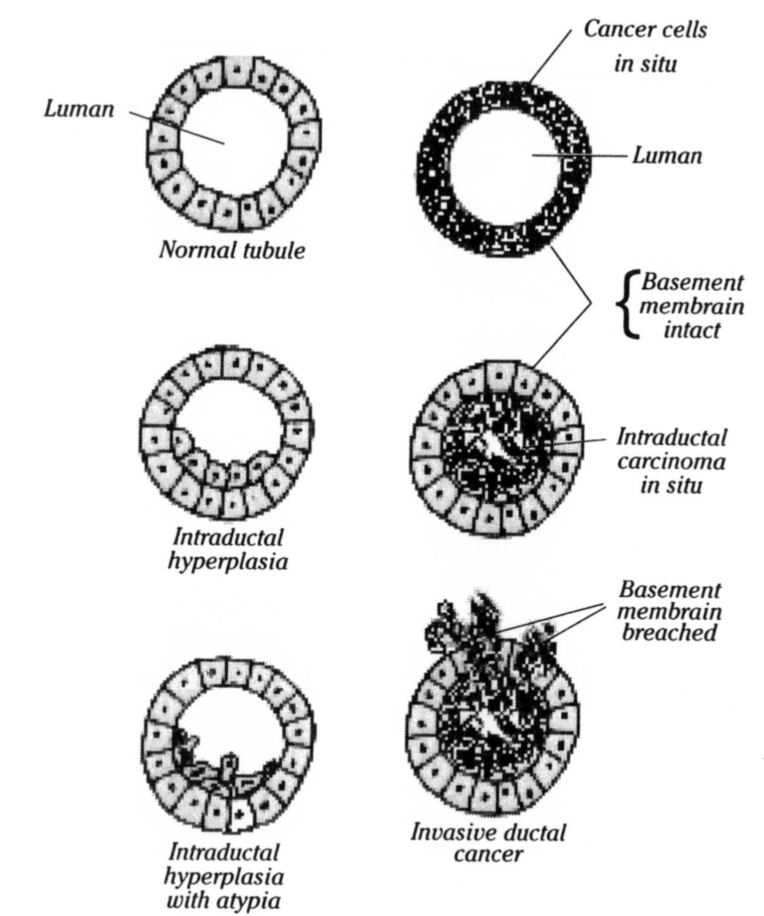
Luman
Normal tubule
Cancer cells
in situ
Luman
Basement
membrain
intact
Intraductal
hyperplasia
Intraductal
carcinoma
in situ
Basement
membrain
breached
Intraductal
hyperplasia
with atypia
Invasive ductal
cancer

Q. What is lobular carcinoma in situ?

A. Lobular carcinoma in situ is not usually detected by mammogram but is found on a breast biopsy performed for other reasons. Its presence is an indication that either the involved breast or the other breast can become malignant. The malignant cells are present in the lobules and terminal ducts in the breast ***(See diagram, p. 5)***. The chance of this cancer spreading into the lymph nodes is 0 percent to 1 percent.

When lobular carcinoma in situ is found, it means that either breast can develop an invasive cancer in the future, and so the treatment recommended is either bilateral mastectomies or close follow-up. Unfortunately, radiation treatment is not very effective in lobular carcinoma in situ. The only good news about this cancer is that it is fairly uncommon: it occurs in less than 10 percent of all of the early cancers that are found.

Women diagnosed with lobular carcinoma in situ have about a 25 percent chance of developing breast cancer during their lifetime.

Q. What are the differences between lobular carcinoma in situ (LCIS) and ductal carcinoma in situ (DCIS)?

A. The following is a table giving some of the differences between lobular carcinoma in situ and ductal carcinoma in situ.

	LCIS	DCIS
PHYSICAL FINDINGS	NONE	NONE, LUMP OR MICROCALCIFICATION
AGE	PREMENOPAUSAL	PRE & POSTMENOPAUSAL
METASTASIS	ALMOST NEVER	OCCASIONAL - Especially when mass present
RISK OF INVASIVE	EITHER BREAST	SAME BREAST - Especially at biopsy site
MAMMOGRAM	NONSPECIFIC	MICROCALCIFICATION OR MASS

Q. **How many doublings (one cell becoming two cells) of breast cancer cells are required to have a tumor 0.5cm or one-fourth inch?**

A. For a tumor to reach the size of one-fourth inch, the cells must have doubled about 27 times.

Q. **At what point in the doubling process does metastasis occur?**

A. Metastasis probably occurs during the first 10 to 20 doublings in the number of cells.

Q. **How fast do breast cancer cells double or divide?**

A. Breast cancer cells do not always divide at the same rate. The cell may not divide for a long time and then suddenly start dividing. The range of cell doubling time has varied between 23 to 209 days with an average of about 100 days.

Q. **How long does it take for one cancer cell to grow to a one-half inch mass?**

A. If one cell divides every 100 days, it will take about eight years for the cancer to grow to a mass one-half inch in size.

Q. **What is Paget's disease of the breast?**

A. Paget's disease is when cancer of the breast, either in situ or invasive, invades the skin of the nipple.

Q. **What is cystosarcoma phyllodes?**

A. This rare tumor is similar to a fibroadenoma; however, the benign type tends to recur. The very rare malignant type can spread to other areas in the body. The usual treatment for the benign type is to keep excising the tumor with a small margin of normal surrounding breast tissue with the hope that it will not recur. If it keeps recurring, a total mastectomy is usually necessary.

Q. **What is infiltrating ductal cancer of the breast?**

A. Infiltrating cancer means that the cancer cells have broken outside of the ducts and have begun invading the other tissue of the breast. If, through a microscope, the pathologist can also see the cancer cells invading blood vessels or lymphatic vessels, it is considered to be more aggressive. Approximately 70 percent to 80 percent of breast cancer is this type of cancer.

Q. **What is inflammatory breast cancer?**

A. Inflammatory breast cancer is a more aggressive breast cancer, making up less than 5 percent of all breast cancers. It develops suddenly, causing the skin of the breast to appear red and infected from cancer cells invading the skin. This type of breast cancer spreads most rapidly.

Q. **Are there any other types of breast cancer?**

A. Some other types of breast cancer include: tubular carcinoma, colloid carcinoma, and papillary carcinoma. These types only occur in 1 percent to 2 percent of women. They've been given these different names because of the appearance of the cells under the microscope. Each of these types of tumors have a slightly better prognosis.

Q. **What is lobular carcinoma?**

A. Lobular carcinoma is a cancer that begins in the lobular epithelium, the location of the cells that manufacture milk. It accounts for approximately 5 percent of all breast cancers. The prognosis for lobular carcinoma is similar to infiltrating duct cell cancer.

Q. What is medullary carcinoma?

A. Medullary carcinoma accounts for less than 5 percent of all breast cancers. Some people believe that the prognosis with medullary carcinoma is slightly better than with other cancers.

Q. I've heard about staging of breast cancer. What does this mean?

A. Staging is when one attempts to categorize how advanced the tumor is. There are two main ways which breast cancer is staged: 1) The TNM parameters, where the T stands for tumor, N for lymph node status, and M for metastasis; and 2) Stages I, II, III, and IV.

The following is a partial explanation of staging:

(Note: One inch = 2.5 cm.)

Tumor

Tx .... The tumor cannot be assessed.
To .... No evidence of tumor.
Tis .... Paget's disease of nipple or carcinoma in situ.
T1 .... Tumor less than 2 cm. in size.
T1a .... Tumor less than 0.5 cm. in size.
T2 .... Tumor larger than 2 cm. but smaller than 5 cm. in size
T3 .... Tumor is greater than 5 cm. in size.
T4 .... Tumor of any size which extends into the chest wall or skin.

Lymph node

Nx .... Original lymph nodes cannot be assessed.
No .... No evidence of lymph node metastasis.
N1 .... Metastasis to same side axillary (armpit) lymph node, moveable.

Metastasis

Mx.............. Presence of metastasis cannot be accessed.
Mo .... No distance of metastasis.
M1.............. Distant metastasis.

The other way to stage breast cancer is the staging system which is as follows:

Stage 0 ...... Carcinoma in situ only.
Stage I .... Tumor less than 2 cm. in size with no evidence of metastasis.
Stage IIa .... Tumor less than 2 cm. in size with metastasis to axillary lymph nodes.
Stage IIb .... Tumor larger than 2 cm. in size with metastasis to axillary lymph nodes.
Stage IIIa ... Tumor of any size with metastasis to lymph nodes which are matted together.
Stage IIIb ... Tumor of any size with extension to the skin and lymph nodes which are matted together.
Stage IV ..... Tumor of any size with or without lymph nodes metastasis, but with distant metastasis present.

Q. **Why is staging of breast cancer necessary?**

A. The staging of breast cancer allows doctors to study the extensiveness of the cancer and to determine both the best type of treatment to use and how well the treatment is working for the tumor, based on the amount of cancer present.

Chapter Eight

BREAST SURGERY FOR CANCER PATIENTS

Q&A

How long have mastectomies been performed?

The ancient Egyptians performed some sort of cauterization (burning) for tumors, and the Romans, before the birth of Christ, surgically removed the breast and some of the chest muscles in breast cancer cases. In the second century, Galen practiced the removal of breast tumors from healthy tissues. In 1162, the Council of Tours recommended non-surgical treatment of breast cancer, and this practice persisted until the end of the Dark Ages when surgical removal was again acceptable. Modern surgery methods did not develop until after anesthesia and antiseptic surgical techniques became widely practiced in the late 1800s.

In 1894, William Halstead described his experience with a radical mastectomy, based on anatomical knowledge of the lymphatic spread of cancer cells. His method included removal of the breast and all the chest wall muscles. This procedure was abandoned in the mid-1970s. D. L. Patey, a British surgeon, is considered the father of current breast cancer surgery. He developed the modified radical mastectomy, first performed in 1932, in which only the breast and the lymph nodes in the armpit are removed. By the mid-1970s, this became the most frequently used operation when American surgeons considered a radical mastectomy to be too much surgery.

Beginning in the 1920s, lumpectomy or partial mastectomy, followed by radiation, was reported sporadically. By the 1970s, multiple reports indicated that radiation treatments after the removal of the tumor were as effective as a mastectomy. Currently, women are given the option of a lumpectomy or a modified radical mastectomy as treatment for early breast cancer.

Q. **What is a lumpectomy?**

A. A lumpectomy means that the entire lump or cancer is removed, along with a rim of normal tissue around the cancer. In addition, a lumpectomy usually means that the patient also has the lower one-third to two-thirds of the lymph nodes under the armpit removed, and she will receive radiation treatment to the breast after surgery.

Q. **What is a modified radical mastectomy?**

A. When a modified radical mastectomy is performed, the entire breast, including the nipple, is removed, along with all the lymph nodes under the armpit. The pectoralis major muscle is not removed, so except for the removal of the breast, there is little defect to the chest wall. This factor makes it possible, in most cases, for a woman to wear a bathing suit without any appearance of abnormality in the upper portion of the chest.

Q. **Is there more than one type of mastectomy?**

A. There are several types of mastectomies: 1) A simple or total mastectomy removes only the breast tissue, leaving the axillary (armpit) nodes intact. 2) A classical radical mastectomy is reserved for very special situations. It requires the removal of the breast and the muscle on the chest wall, as well as the lymph nodes under the arm. This is the most disfiguring type of operation, and the one that women have feared most in the past because it leaves an indentation under the clavicle or collar bone. 3) A modified radical mastectomy removes the entire breast, along with all of the axillary lymph nodes, but it does not cause any indentation under the clavicle because the pectoralis muscle is not removed. 4) A lumpectomy or partial mastectomy removes only the cancer, along with a rim of normal breast which surrounds the cancer. Radiation treatment begins about three weeks after the surgery.

Q. **Before I have either a lumpectomy or mastectomy, what pre-operative tests is the surgeon likely to conduct?**

A. Pre-operative tests are used to determine if there is any evidence of the spread of cancer and to determine a base line for evaluation and follow-up after surgery. Pre-operative tests usually include a chest X-ray. Some physicians include a bone and liver scan or recommend certain blood studies consisting of CEA, CA15-3, and CA549 (proteins which are sometimes found in the blood with breast cancer). The problems with these blood tests for cancer are that they are not very reliable and are mainly used experimentally.

It is important that you have a mammogram before you have surgery for breast cancer. The mammogram should include both breasts to make sure that 1) there is no cancer in the other breast, and 2) there is no additional cancer in the involved breast.

Q. **If I have a breast biopsy and am found to have cancer, how important is it that I not delay further treatment or surgery?**

A. This question has never been fully answered. There have been a number of retrospective studies, however, that indicate waiting several weeks does not seem to make any difference in the chance of being cured. But take note: once a cancer can be felt, it probably has been present several years prior to the biopsy, so if the cancer was going to spread, a delay of several weeks probably would not be harmful.

Q. **If a biopsy shows that I have breast cancer, will the surgeon do an immediate mastectomy or lumpectomy and axillary dissection (removal of armpit nodes)?**

A. Surgeons seldom recommend a single step procedure for breast cancer treatment. Ideally, every woman should have some time to think about the treatment options after a biopsy is performed. A biopsy can, of course, sometimes be performed with a needle in a physician's office, so only one operation is needed if cancer is found. After the biopsy, the patient can get an opinion from a radiation therapist or plastic surgeon to see if something other than a total mastectomy is appropriate. If the patient has already made up her mind about the type of treatment she wants, there is no problem with immediate surgical treatment after a biopsy, if the surgeon agrees with this plan.

Q. **When did lumpectomy and radiation gain wide acceptance and popularity?**

A. In the 1960s surgeons began performing partial mastectomies and radiation therapy with some regularity. By the 1970s, it was becoming obvious that radiation and a lumpectomy or partial mastectomy gave results similar to those attained by a modified radical mastectomy. It was not until the 1980s that the general medical community became convinced that many women could be effectively treated for breast cancer with less surgery than a total mastectomy.

Q. **If I have breast cancer, what treatment will give me the best results: a modified radical mastectomy or a lumpectomy and radiation?**

A. This is the question most frequently asked by women who discover they have breast cancer. The answer is that the long term survival is essentially the same if the women undergoing a lumpectomy and radiation meet the necessary criteria for this procedure. About 80 percent of breast cancer patients are potential candidates for a breast-conserving procedure, which means they would undergo a lumpectomy and the removal of lymph nodes, followed by radiation treatment.

OPTIONS FOR EARLY BREAST CANCER TREATMENT
(if less than 50 years of age and still having menstrual periods)

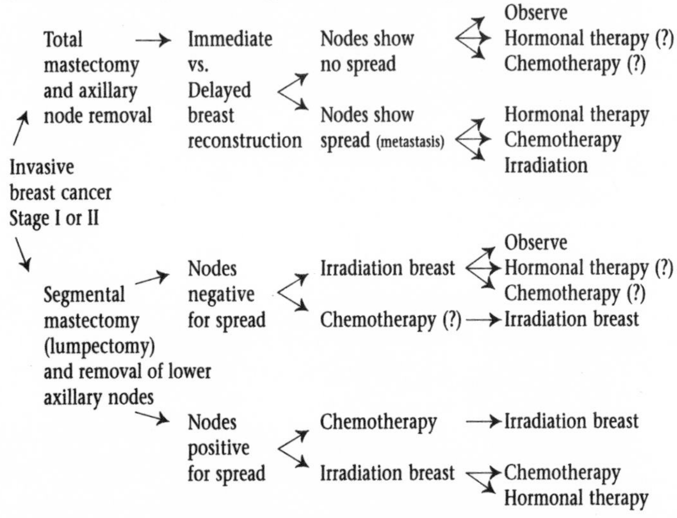

Q. **What type of patient would and would not be a candidate for lumpectomy surgery and radiation?**

A. The patient's tumor should be small enough so that once it is removed, along with approximately one-half-inch margin of normal tissue around the tumor, the cosmetic result would not be disfiguring.

If a woman has a breast tumor located directly underneath the nipple, she would be a candidate for a lumpectomy and radiation, but may require the removal of the nipple.

A woman whose tumors are located in multiple areas of the breast is not a good candidate. Pregnancy also disqualifies a patient from this procedure because the necessary follow-up radiation treatments would be harmful to a woman's developing baby.

A woman who has undergone radiation for another problem in the chest area may not be able to have a lumpectomy because it requires additional radiation which would be harmful to her.

If a patient is not able to undergo the inconvenience of travel to the hospital for daily radiation treatments five times per week, for six weeks, she should consider another form of treatment for breast cancer.

Q. **Is it absolutely necessary for me to receive radiation to my breast after a lumpectomy?**

A. Yes. About 40 percent of women will eventually develop recurrent cancer in the breast after a lumpectomy if they do NOT receive radiation. Unfortunately, there is no way to determine which women are in this 40 percent group, so as a preventive measure, radiation is recommended for all women who have undergone a lumpectomy.

Q. **Which is more difficult for a surgeon: a modified radical mastectomy or a lumpectomy?**

A. A lumpectomy is more difficult because the lymph nodes are removed through a smaller cosmetic incision under the armpit.

Q. **What is the average hospital stay for a mastectomy? A lumpectomy?**

A. Today, mastectomy patients spend one to three nights in the hospital. Patients who have undergone lumpectomy surgery, including lymph node removal, may go home the day of surgery or the next day.

Q. **A friend of mine had to have two lumpectomies before she underwent radiation treatment for breast cancer. Why would she need two lumpectomies before radiation treatment?**

A. In a lumpectomy approach to treatment, the most important thing is to make sure that all of the tumor has been removed before the breast is radiated. In order to do this, at least one-half inch of normal breast tissue must be removed around any tumor tissue. The pathologist usually needs a couple of days to process the tissue and then examine it. If all the tumor was not removed in the first lumpectomy, a second lumpectomy would be necessary.

Q. **If a malignant tumor has been removed with a lumpectomy, why would it be necessary to remove the whole breast, or to follow-up the lumpectomy with radiation treatments?**

A. As already stated, malignancies recur in approximately 40 percent of the cases of breast cancer when the treatment has been limited to removal of the tumor only without follow-up radiation or removal of the whole breast. Because it is impossible to know which women will comprise that 40 percent, all breast cancer patients need to be treated with these additional preventive procedures. Breast cancer tumors can recur if cancer cells remain in the breast and then later re-grow.

Q. **If I have a lumpectomy, why do the lymph nodes have to be removed?**

A. Lymph nodes are removed and evaluated to determine the stage of the cancer and the need for chemotherapy. The lymph nodes are also removed so that they will not have to be irradiated or surgically removed later if the tumor in the lymph nodes grows. Radiation therapists generally do not like to radiate the lymph nodes because radiation can cause the arm to swell.

Q. **What would happen if the cancer recurred in my breast after it had been treated with a lumpectomy and radiation?**

A. The overall chance of this happening is about 5 percent, but if it occurred, a mastectomy generally would have to be performed.

Q. **Are as many lymph nodes removed with lumpectomy surgery as with a modified radical mastectomy?**

A. No. In a lumpectomy surgery with an axillary dissection (surgical removal of the lymph nodes), only the lower one-third to two-thirds of the lymph nodes are removed. When a modified mastectomy is performed, all the lymph nodes in the armpit are removed.

Q. **At the time of my lumpectomy or mastectomy, can you simply check my lymph nodes and not remove them all?**

A. It is very difficult to individually inspect and remove lymph nodes in the armpit or axilla because they are imbedded in fat and are difficult to find.

Q. **If only the lower two-thirds of lymph nodes are removed with a lumpectomy, how will I know that the cancer could not have spread to the other lymph nodes which were not removed?**

A. According to studies, in only about 2 percent to 3 percent of cases does the cancer spread to the upper one-third of the lymph nodes which were *not* removed. This small chance of missing the spread of the cancer is not considered great enough to risk other complications that arise from removing all the lymph nodes—complications such as arm and breast edema (swelling) and possible injury to the cutaneous nerve which gives sensation to the inner upper arm.

Q. **If the surgeon removes two-thirds of my axillary (armpit) nodes and leaves one or two nodes which have cancer in them, will this affect me in the future?**

A. Studies on this question have yielded unclear results. Dr. Bernard Fisher, a pioneer in breast conservation for breast cancer, has shown this does not have any adverse effect on the death rate of breast cancer.

Q. **If I have lumpectomy surgery, will my arm be numb on the inside like my neighbor's, who had a modified radical mastectomy?**

A. When a surgeon performs an axillary sampling with lumpectomy surgery, sometimes the small sensory nerve which supplies feeling to the inner skin of the upper arm is cut. Some surgeons will try to save this nerve, if at all possible, and you should certainly ask them to try. However, even if the nerve cannot be saved, it would be unusual if you experienced any long term problems and, in fact, you can expect some feeling in the inner arm to return in time.

Q. **What are the advantages of a modified radical mastectomy?**

A. Modified radical mastectomy is the gold standard to which all other breast cancer surgeries are compared. A modified radical mastectomy removes the breast and all of the cancer, as well as the axillary (armpit) lymph nodes, and yields less chance of recurrence of cancer on the chest where the breast used to be. Psychologically, some women prefer this surgery because it removes the tissue which they consider to be a threat to them.

Q. **What are the disadvantages of a modified radical mastectomy?**

A. The main disadvantage is, of course, cosmetic. The other disadvantages are that the arm will most likely be numb on the inside of the upper arm because the sensory nerve is generally removed. The skin where the breast was removed is also numb. About 5 percent of the time, healing problems occur on the skin on the chest wall. Sometimes scar tissue on the chest wall and in the armpit will cause a woman to have difficulty regaining her normal range of arm motion.

Q. **If I have cancer in my lymph nodes, is it better to surgically remove them, or to treat the cancer with radiation?**

A. With both treatments, the survival rates are about the same, and complications such as arm swelling are comparable—about 5 percent to 7 percent of the time. If complete surgical removal of the lymph nodes is followed by radiation treatments to the armpit, the incidence of edema (swelling of the arm) goes up because the radiation causes additional scarring in the tissue. If only a portion of the lymph nodes are removed, as in a lumpectomy, the chance of arm swelling is reduced. In general, it is better to surgically remove the lymph nodes than to treat them with radiation because all the lymph nodes can then be examined microscopically by the pathologist.

Q. **If the lymph nodes under my arm are removed, are there any special concerns I should know about?**

A. Yes. Infection and swelling of the arm are the two main concerns. Infection in the arm can spread much more rapidly because the lymph nodes are no longer present to trap bacteria. Special care should be taken to prevent any cuts or injury to the involved arm. Repeat infections can cause injury to the remaining lymph nodes and lymphatics in the arm, and this increases the possibility of the arm swelling. Taking antibiotics at the first sign of any infection in the arm may be helpful in preventing a more serious infection.

Q. **If I have edema (swelling) of my arm, what can I do for relief?**

A. First, lean women have less swelling, so if you are lean, avoid gaining extra weight. Elevating your arm, massaging it, and wearing medically designed, tight-fitting gloves and sleeves control most edema. If the condition worsens, an apparatus called a pneumatic compressive pump can be used to decrease the swelling.

Q. **What about exercises after a mastectomy or lumpectomy?**

A. Doing exercises after a mastectomy or lumpectomy prevents the shoulder from becoming painful and stiff. The exercises are intended to stretch the developing scar tissue and to keep it soft and pliable, helping you to regain full use of your arm as soon as possible. In most cases, your surgeon will allow you to begin exercising within three weeks after surgery, if the tissues are adequately healed.

The exercises, best taught by volunteers from the Reach For Recovery organization, include exercises that will help you straighten and raise your arm, allowing you to be able to reach above your head with normal mobility. Squeezing a rubber ball is used to milk out any swelling in the arm. Stretching exercises also make the arm less painful and improve a woman's posture after a mastectomy.

Q. **When can I start wearing a prosthesis after my mastectomy?**

A. Most women can wear a temporary prosthesis and bra when they leave the hospital. A Reach for Recovery volunteer is usually available at this time and will provide a soft, cotton, fluff-like prosthesis that does not put any pressure on the healing wound. After three weeks, a woman can usually wear a more permanent prosthesis. These prostheses are usually made of a soft gel material and come in many shapes and sizes. The Reach for Recovery volunteer or your doctor's office can give you information on where to buy one. The cost of a prosthesis can be as much as three hundred dollars, but most are covered by insurance.

Q. **Do I have to have a mastectomy if I only have ductal cell carcinoma?**

A. The preferred treatment for ductal cell carcinoma in situ is not known at present. Studies show that in some women, if the tumor is only one-half inch in size, removal of the tumor is sufficient, and no further treatment is necessary. However, this has been shown only for ductal cell carcinomas in situ that are slow growing. These slow growing tumors do not have dead cells in the ducts, nor do they have a high nuclear grade or rate of division (S phase).

The type of ductal carcinoma in situ which has a much higher recurrence rate is called comedo carcinoma in situ, and this type seems to have a much greater chance of recurrence if it is simply removed. Approximately half the time, this type of tumor will come back as invasive cancer and can spread. Studies show, however, that radiation treatment for ductal carcinoma in situ decreases the chance of it recurring; studies also show that the recurrence of cancer in the breast is slightly higher than the recurrence seen when radiation is used to treat an invasive cancer. Most physicians believe patients having a ductal cell carcinoma in situ that is two to three inches in size or greater probably should have the lower armpit lymph nodes removed, because there is a 2 percent to 3 percent chance that it may spread to these lymph nodes. If the tumor is smaller than this, the chance of it spreading to the lymph is quite remote.

Even with all the above information, physicians are not certain whether the best treatment for ductal carcinoma in situ is either simply excision of only the tumor in special cases, radiation treatment after excision, or a mastectomy. Also complicating the data is the fact that the incidence of ductal carcinoma in situ is increasing because it is being found more frequently by mammograms. Studies have also revealed that in many instances, women who discovered they had ductal carcinoma in situ did not eventually develop invasive breast cancer. Fortunately, there are several trials going on right now to find out what is the best treatment for ductal carcinoma in situ.

One thing we do know for certain is this: If a woman has a mastectomy as treatment for ductal carcinoma in situ, and if there is no evidence of the cancer having spread to the lymph nodes, the chance of her being cured is 99 percent. For this reason, many women choose a mastectomy to treat this very early type of breast cancer.

OPTIONS FOR TREATMENT OF DUCTAL CARCINOMA IN SITU (DCIS)

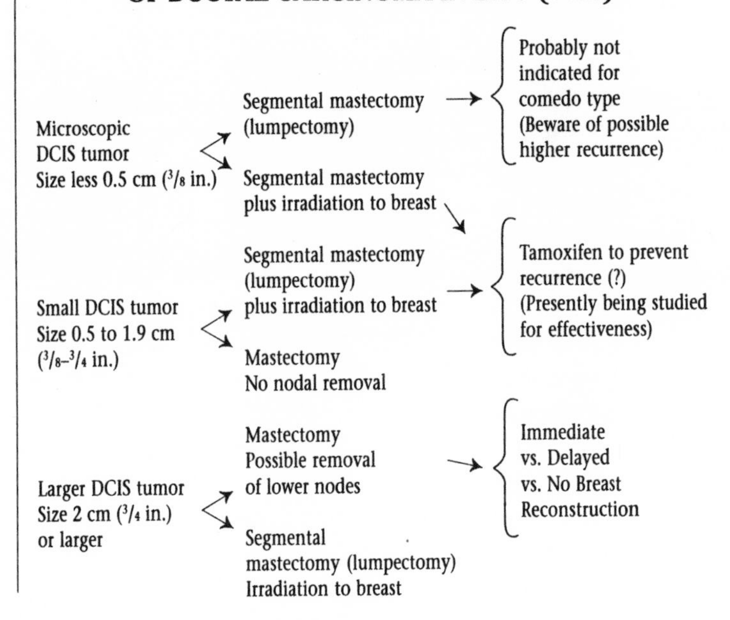

Q. **I have a friend who was found to have lobular carcinoma in situ in one breast. They removed both of her breasts. Is this the normal treatment for this type of cancer which has not spread out of the ducts?**

A. Lobular carcinoma in situ is mainly an indicator that a woman has a 25 percent-*plus* chance of developing an invasive cancer in either breast over the next 20 years of her life. Because of this very high chance of developing an invasive breast cancer in either breast, some surgeons have recommended that both breasts be removed. If both breasts are not removed, then the patient must be very committed to frequent and thorough follow-up physical examinations and mammograms.

A few surgeons are recommending removal of the breast in which the cancer was found, and then performing a biopsy on the other breast in the same area. If a lobular carcinoma is found in the other breast, then it too would be removed. If this treatment is done, the woman must still understand that she probably has a 25 percent-plus chance of developing breast cancer in the remaining breast over the next 20 years of her life.

Q. **If I have a scoop-out procedure or subcutaneous mastectomy in which they remove my breast tissue but not my nipple and skin, will that prevent me from developing breast cancer in the future?**

A. A subcutaneous mastectomy in which the nipple and the skin is left behind does not provide total prevention for any future cancer. This is because it is very difficult to remove all of the breast tissue, especially the breast tissue connected to the nipple. It is true that a decrease in the volume of the breast tissue may decrease the chances of one developing future breast cancer, as some have suggested, but it is not a certainty, because some breast tissue still remains.

The cosmetic result from a subcutaneous mastectomy leaves a woman completely flat, making an implant necessary. (Implants covered by only a thin layer of skin do not give a good cosmetic result.)

Q. **If I have had one breast removed for invasive breast cancer, should I have a prophylactic mastectomy on my remaining breast?**

A. The chance of developing cancer in the remaining breast is slightly less than 1 percent a year. With the chance being this low, most women do not elect to have their remaining breast removed. A prophylactic mastectomy might be recommended if a patient had a family history of breast cancer that included a genetic potential for bilateral cancer, or if the tumor was intraductal lobular carcinoma, which has a high incidence of either breast developing invasive cancer. Plastic surgeons will sometimes favor removing the other breast or reducing its size if it is large and will be difficult to match with reconstruction. Many insurance companies, however, will not pay for a prophylactic mastectomy.

Chapter Nine

RADIATION CANCER TREATMENT

Q. **Why is radiation used to treat breast cancer?**

A. Radiation treatment for breast cancer has been employed for about fifty years and it is used because breast cancer tumors are sensitive to the effects of radiation. In fact, breast cancer tumor cells are more sensitive to radiation than are the normal cells within the body. For this reason, the radiation has a greater effect on breast cancer than on the normal breast tissue. The course of radiation treatments used in breast cancer is designed to, ideally, leave no breast cancer cells alive at the end of the course of radiation, while at the same time having little or no impact on the normal tissues of the breast.

Q. **How is radiation given to the patient?**

A. When undergoing radiation treatment, the patient lies on a table in "treatment position," that is, lying with the arm on the side of the breast cancer positioned at a 90-degree angle from the body. Highly sophisticated radiation treatment machines are used to deliver the radiation treatments in a very precise fashion. The two most common forms of treatment machines are a cobalt unit or a linear accelerator. The patient is in the treatment room for about twenty minutes, but the actual treatment itself takes only a couple of minutes. The majority of the time in the treatment room involves positioning the patient correctly so that the treatments can be delivered accurately.

Q. **How much radiation is given to the breast?**

A. The entire breast receives 4500 to 5000 rad or cGy over a five-week period, with treatments given five days a week. In most cases, this course of treatment is then followed by a "boost" treatment. This means the patient receives an additional 1000 rad in five treatment days, and the radiation is directed only around the breast scar in the area of the original site of the primary breast cancer. The "boost" of radiation may also be administered by placing radioactive tubes close to the site of the original cancer.

Q. **How does the radiation received during treatment compare to other radiation we receive, for instance, while getting a chest X-ray?**

A. The radiation exposure in a chest X-ray is spread out over a large surface and is used for diagnostic purposes, to obtain a picture of what things look like within the chest cavity. Radiation exposure during breast cancer treatment directs the radiation onto a much smaller area, using very refined and exact methods which prevent other areas of the body from being affected.

Q. **What are the harmful effects of radiation?**

A. The tissues that are affected the most by the radiation are the cancer cells, *not* the normal cells of the body. The normal, healthy body cells are able to repair themselves after radiation exposure, but the cancer cells, which are abnormal, cannot repair themselves as easily. This, of course, is the goal of radiation treatment—the destruction of the cancerous cells.

Radiation treatments may cause a patient's skin to become irritated and to appear tanned. However, within three to four weeks after completing radiation treatment, these conditions usually disappear. In some instances, swelling of the breast tissue will occur during the course of radiation treatment, but this is not considered a serious medical problem. The swelling usually goes away within a few weeks, sometimes months, after the cancer treatment is finished. It is unusual for a patient to suffer any lasting cosmetic effects from radiation treatment to the breast.

Q. **Will I have any nausea or other problems while I am undergoing radiation treatment?**

A. Undergoing a radiation treatment is much like getting a chest X-ray: you will feel *no* immediate effects, such as nausea or light-headedness. You can expect to be able to carry out your normal activities throughout the duration of your treatments. You can drive yourself to and from the treatment center. If you do experience any side effects during the course of your treatment, such as the skin irritation mentioned above, these will not appear until the third or fourth week of treatment. But remember, this condition and the others already discussed usually disappear within three to four weeks after your treatments have been completed.

Q. **What will my breast look like while I am receiving radiation?**

A. The skin of your breast may become irritated or tan-looking sometime during the third or fourth week of your treatment. It is unusual for the treatment to cause blisters. Slight swelling of the breast may occur during the course of the radiation treatments, but again, this is usually resolved soon after the treatment is completed.

Q. **What are the long-term effects of radiation on my breast?**

A. There are usually no long-term effects of radiation treatments. The skin reactions and the swelling described above can be expected to clear up within three to four weeks after your last radiation treatment. Sometimes breast tissue is tender for several weeks after radiation treatment, but this is not a common condition. Women are not able to breast-feed with the treated breast after radiation treatments.

Q. **Will radiation burn my skin?**

A. Today, most cancer treatment facilities use modern equipment and state-of-the-art technology, which means patients receiving radiation treatment should have little reason to worry about being burned. Only rarely does radiation produce a significant skin reaction, and when it does occur, the condition clears shortly after the treatments end.

Q. **Can radiation treatments cause me to develop new cancers or cancers of the other breast?**

A. Radiation exposure can always put one at risk of developing a new cancer; however, the risk of this happening is extremely small. Risk of cancers of the other breast probably is not increased.

Q. **What type of patient is the best candidate for radiation treatments?**

A. This depends on two factors: the type of surgery the breast cancer patient has undergone and the pathological features of the tumor removed. All patients that have undergone lumpectomy treatment are automatically candidates for radiation treatments to the remaining breast tissue. In these cases, the radiation treatment provides the same protection that a modified radical mastectomy would give the patient. A lumpectomy combined with radiation treatment is an appropriate choice for patients whose cancerous breast tumors are small, whose tumors were confined to the breast, or whose tumors showed only early signs of spreading to the axillary (armpit) lymph nodes.

Q. **What type of patient cannot receive radiation treatments to the breast?**

A. There are few patients who are *not* candidates for radiation treatments for early breast cancer. Occasionally, we will see a patient with such large breasts that it becomes technically difficult to deliver the radiation treatments. It also happens that women with very small breasts often have little or no breast left for radiation if an extremely large tumor has been removed. In addition, physicians recommend that patients with lupus or scleroderma not undergo long courses of radiation treatment.

Q. **How does breast size affect radiation treatment?**

A. Patients with large breasts are at more risk of developing swelling of the breasts during and after completion of the treatments. Again, this is usually a short term condition, going away within weeks after treatment is completed. Patients with large breasts are also at a higher risk of developing a more intense skin reaction.

Q. **Does it make any difference if I have small breasts?**

A. Small breasts do not make any difference in the treatment approach with radiation, provided an adequate margin of normal breast tissue can be removed surgically from around the cancer without disfiguring the breast.

Q. **How do radiation oncologists know where on the breast to direct the radiation?**

A. Radiation oncologists are expertly trained in all aspects of radiation, and the technical parameters of radiation placement are well-defined. Generally speaking, however, most of the breast tissue is included in the treatment field, with special care taken to be sure the lungs, heart, and bones receive little or no radiation.

Q. **Will radiation affect movement of my arm?**

A. Radiation will *not* in any way affect the movement of your arm.

Q. **What is the chance of the cancer coming back in my irradiated breast?**

A. If all the microscopic and palpable cancer is removed by the surgeon at the time of the lumpectomy, and if this surgery is then followed by a course of radiation treatments, there is a less than 10 percent chance of the cancer returning within the breast tissue.

Q. **Are there instances when radiation cannot be used for breast cancer?**

A. The use of radiation in the treatment of breast cancer is usually a matter of timing. For instance, if the patient's breast cancer was in an advanced stage, treatment would not begin with radiation treatment. Instead, the patient would undergo several cycles of chemotherapy and have surgery before she would undergo radiation treatments.

Treatment of carcinoma of the breast is a highly individualized situation, and the sequence of surgery, radiation treatments, and chemotherapy may vary from patient to patient.

Q. **What happens if the cancer returns in my irradiated breast?**

A. In most cases, the patient will undergo a mastectomy, which usually yields good results. However, researchers are conducting studies to determine if the simple removal of the recurrent cancer is adequate in cases where the recurrent cancer is one-half inch in size, or less.

Q. **How would I know if the cancer has recurred in my irradiated breast?**

A. A breast cancer patient continues to be monitored by either her family physician or her surgeon after completing all her cancer treatments. She undergoes physical exams as well as mammograms on a regular basis, and any recurrence of her cancer can be quickly discovered in this way. If the cancer is going to recur in the breast, it will usually recur within three years.

Q. **If I choose to undergo a modified radical mastectomy as treatment for my breast cancer, will I ever need radiation treatments after the mastectomy?**

A. If the pathologist's report on the tumor shows that the cancer has certain aggressive features that would put the patient at risk of a cancer recurring on the chest wall, then yes, radiation treatments would be necessary. Also, if the tumor was very large, greater than two inches, and had spread to many axillary (armpit) lymph nodes, then radiation would be used to prevent the cancer from recurring on the skin of the chest.

Q. **If my breast cancer spreads to another part of my body, can radiation treatments be used?**

A. Yes. Radiation treatments are very effective in treating the metastatic spread of breast cancer tumors and can greatly improve the patient's quality of life.

Q. **Can I receive radiation if I am pregnant?**

A. We prefer not to give radiation until after the baby is born because there is a small risk of radiation injuring the developing baby. Unfortunately, the baby can not be completely shielded from the radiation.

Q. **Will I be able to breast-feed after I receive radiation to my breast?**

A. Women are not able to breast-feed with the treated breast after radiation treatments.

Chapter Ten

DRUG TREATMENT FOR BREAST CANCER

Q. Why give any type of chemotherapy or drug treatment for breast cancer?

A. Chemotherapy is recommended for the treatment of breast cancer either to improve the quality of life or to extend life. When chemotherapy is given after surgery for breast cancer, it is called adjuvant treatment. Adjuvant chemotherapy helps reduce the chance that the breast cancer will recur by killing any cancer cells that may still remain. When breast cancer develops, the cancer cells often quickly acquire the ability to move outside the breast. Since cancer cells that have migrated elsewhere are small, they are called micrometastases and are undetectable by any blood test or X-ray exam.

Q. **What type of physician specializes in chemotherapy?**

A. A medical oncologist is a physician who has first completed three years of training in internal medicine. To specialize in the diagnosis and medical treatment of cancer, another two to three years of training is required for certification as a medical oncologist.

Q. **How does chemotherapy work?**

A. Chemotherapy works by interfering with the normal growth of cancer cells, usually by disrupting important cellular processes. Some drugs, called alkylating agents, prevent DNA replication, while others, the antimetabolites, interfere with enzymes needed for cell division.

Q. What are the most common side effects of chemotherapy?

A. Nausea, loss of appetite, vomiting, hair loss, fatigue, and low blood counts are the more common side effects. The frequency and severity of these side effects varies greatly depending on the individual. Treatment toxicities also depend on the amount of drug prescribed, the method of administration, and the specific drug.

Q. Why does chemotherapy cause side effects?

A. Chemotherapy has an effect on all cells that are actively growing. This includes tumor cells that divide quickly and normal body cells which also divide quickly, such as cells of the gastrointestinal tract, the bone marrow, and hair cells.

Q. How many drugs are given with adjuvant chemotherapy?

A. The most common treatment regimens include three different medications. The drug combinations are chosen to avoid overlapping side effects and to take advantage of the different mechanisms of action of each drug. Using combinations of drugs also may reduce the development of tumor resistance to a specific drug.

Q. After breast cancer surgery, when is the best time to begin adjuvant chemotherapy?

A. Adjuvant chemotherapy is usually started four to six weeks after breast surgery. These few weeks allow the patient to recover from the operation and provide time for the tissue to heal.

Q. How long does adjuvant treatment last?

A. Adjuvant chemotherapy is given every three to four weeks for a total of six courses, approximately 18 to 24 weeks. If hormonal therapy is advised, current recommendations are to continue tamoxifen for at least two to five years.

Q. **Which chemotherapy drugs are used most often?**

A. The most commonly used treatment regimens are "FAC" and "CMF." FAC is an abbreviation for fluorouracil, doxorubicin, and cyclophosphamide. CMF includes the drugs cyclophosphamide, methotrexate, and fluorouracil. Each of these treatment regimens is given as an outpatient and repeated at three- to four-week intervals for a total of six cycles.

Q. **How do I know if the chemotherapy is working?**

A. The answer is that we don't know if the desired effect of treatment (no cancer recurrence) will occur. In fact, therapy is started when there is no evidence of disease anywhere. Similarly, during chemotherapy and afterwards, there are no specific tests that will tell us if all the cancer cells have been eradicated.

Q. **Is there a chance that the cancer could still come back even after I've taken chemotherapy?**

A. Yes, chemotherapy treatment does not reduce the risk of recurrence to zero. There are several possibilities for why chemotherapy is not 100 percent effective. Each dose of chemotherapy kills a certain fraction of the tumor cells, depending on the dose given. Often, the remaining cells develop a resistance to the actions of the chemotherapy drugs. Eventually, these resistant cells grow and are insensitive to the toxic effects of chemotherapy.

Q. **I have heard there is another type of drug therapy for treating breast cancer, in addition to chemotherapy.**

A. Chemotherapy refers to drugs that have a direct anti-cancer effect on malignant cells. Another effective type of therapy for breast cancer is hormonal therapy. Hormone therapy uses medications that block the normal actions of the female hormones, estrogen and progesterone. The most common hormonal agent is tamoxifen; Nolvadex is the trade name. Tamoxifen, an anti-estrogen, attaches to cell surface proteins that normally combine with estrogen, thus blocking the action of estrogen on cancer cells and preventing cell growth. Hormone therapy does not directly kill cancer cells.

Q. **Are there other hormonal agents, besides tamoxifen, that are used to treat breast cancer?**

A. Progesterone, high-dose estrogens, and other hormones also are effective when treating metastatic or advanced breast cancer. They have not been used as adjuvant hormone therapy, partly because tamoxifen has so few side effects. In the adjuvant setting, there are non-medical ways to reduce the risk of recurrent breast cancer. We know that survival in young women is improved when normal levels of estrogen are decreased, either by surgically removing the ovaries or giving radiation to the ovaries.

Q. **Are there many side effects with tamoxifen?**

A. Tamoxifen has few side effects and women seldom have to stop treatment for drug-related toxicities. The most common problem is hot flashes similar to those that occur with menopause. These are more prominent in younger women than in older women. Other side effects include vaginal discharge, nausea, and depression although they appear in less than 5 percent of women on the drug.

Tamoxifen is not a “pure” anti-estrogen; it has weak estrogen-like effects on some tissues of the body. These estrogen-like effects may be beneficial. If taking tamoxifen, the normal bone loss that occurs with age is slowed and total cholesterol levels are lower.

Q. **I've read that tamoxifen can cause uterine cancer.**

A. A few studies have detected slightly more cases of endometrial (uterine) cancer than expected in women taking tamoxifen. This may be related to the estrogen-like properties of the drug. Uterine cancer, however, is not difficult to diagnose and is easily treated with surgery. Concern about this low possibility should not prevent you from taking tamoxifen if it is recommended.

Q. **Who should receive chemotherapy?**

A. This question generates much debate. Most oncologists would advise treatment if the woman has at least a 25 percent to 30 percent chance of having the cancer return; however, many others feel that women with a much lower chance of recurrence should also receive treatment. I feel a woman should get all the information she can that will give her the best estimate of her chances of developing recurrent cancer, and then she should make the decision after she has weighed all the risks and benefits of chemotherapy.

Q. **What information is used to decide if chemotherapy is indicated?**

A. The most important features of early breast cancer that determine prognosis are the size of the cancer and the presence or absence of tumor cells in the lymph nodes. Physicians use tumor size and node involvement plus other prognostic factors to make decisions about adjuvant therapy. Prognostic factors help to separate women into low-risk and high-risk groups in terms of probability of breast cancer recurrence. Women at very low-risk for recurrence should be spared the toxicity and expense of treatment, and those women at high-risk should be advised about the benefits of adjuvant treatment.

Here is an example of how nodal involvement indicates the chance of recurrence of cancer. The following survival numbers are approximate:

Number of nodes	***Survival at 5 years***
0	*83 %*
1	*80 %*
3	*70 %*
4	*47 %*
13 or more	*28 %*

Here is an example of how tumor size with *no* spread to the lymph nodes affects outcome. The following survival numbers are approximate:

Size of tumor	***Survival at 5 years***
less than .40 inch	*98 %*
.40 to 1.25 inch	*91 %*
larger 1.25 inch	*85 %*

Here is an example showing that the likelihood that lymph nodes will contain cancer increases as the size of the breast tumor increases. The following numbers are approximate:

Tumor size	***Percent with positive nodes***
less 0.40 inch	*20 %*
.40 to .75 inch	*33 %*
.75 to 1.12 inch	*45 %*
1.12 to 1.5 inch	*50 %*
1.5 to 2.0 inch	*60 %*
larger than 2 inches	*70 %*

Q. **Do I need a bone scan before or after my surgery?**

A. The use of bone scans if no bone pain is present is controversial. Bone scans are usually too sensitive to differentiate between degenerative (arthritic) joint disease and cancer, resulting in a positive bone scan although no cancer is present in the bone. Also, the time lapse is usually brief between a positive bone scan finding and the development of bone pain (indicating cancer), thereby providing little, if any, real benefit, since it is debated whether earlier treatment of cancer that has spread to the bone improves the chances of survival. Some physicians will obtain a bone scan only when the initial stage of the cancer is more advanced to obtain a baseline study for comparison with future scans should the patient ever develop bone pain.

Q. **How often do I need a chest X-ray after breast cancer?**

A. Unfortunately, there is no proof that obtaining routine, post-treatment chest X-rays improves survival.

Q. **Do I need any liver tests before or after my surgery?**

A. Routine liver evaluations with ultrasound, nuclear scans, MRI and CAT scans have not been useful in detecting cancer spread if the patient has no symptoms and the blood does not show any abnormal liver changes. Some physicians will obtain such studies for a baseline if they feel there is a higher than usual chance that the cancer has spread to the liver.

Q. **Are there other characteristics of the tumor that help determine prognosis?**

A. Other standard prognostic features are available after the tumor is removed and studied in the laboratory, as illustrated in the following chart:

CHARACTERISTIC	FAVORABLE	UNFAVORABLE
Pathological inflammatory breast cancer	ductal carcinoma in situ	
classification	tubular cancer	
histologic grade	well differentiated	poorly differentiated
Estrogen and progesterone receptor status	positive and high	negative or low
Tumor growth rate S-phase fraction (S= synthesis)	low	high
Tumor DNA content	normal	abnormal
Experimental measures		
Her-2/neu gene	not elevated	elevated
Cathepsin-D	not elevated	elevated

Q. **Are considerations of chemotherapy or hormonal therapy different for premenopausal and postmenopausal women?**

A. Clinical trials show that chemotherapy is more effective in premenopausal women. With no involved nodes, premenopausal women can expect approximately a 36-percent odds' reduction for the risk of recurrent cancer. The risk reduction for postmenopausal women who receive chemotherapy is less, approximately 27 percent.

In contrast, tamoxifen is more effective in postmenopausal women, especially those with involved nodes and positive estrogen receptor values. Hormonal therapy is not as effective in premenopausal women because more of the tumors are unresponsive to hormones. This is probably because young women have high estrogen levels.

Q. **What is meant by a relative reduction in cancer recurrence if I take chemotherapy? I thought chemotherapy helps everyone who takes it.**

A. Chemotherapy does *not* help *all* of the patients who take it for two main reasons: First, surgery or radiation may cure the cancer and it will not reoccur whether one does or does not take chemotherapy. Second, the chemotherapy does not have an effect on the cancer cells of *all* the patients who will develop a recurrent cancer. An example of this fact can be illustrated using two sets of patients, 100 patients in each set, assuming that the chemotherapy has a 30 percent relative reduction in recurrence of cancer.

Low risk group:
The low risk group has only a 10-percent chance of the cancer recurring without any further treatment, since 90 percent will be cured with surgery or radiation. If this 100 patients take the chemotherapy, then only 3 of the 10 patients who will develop a recurrence will be helped. In other words, 97 percent of the patients will take the chemotherapy and get *no* benefit from the drugs.

High risk group:
The high risk group has a 40-percent chance of the cancer recurring without any further treatment. If all 100 patients take chemotherapy, then 12 patients, or 12 percent, will benefit from the treatment. The other 88 percent gain nothing from the drugs.

Q. **What are the many factors that predict developing recurrent cancer in a stage I or II breast cancer patient?**

A. The following table presents the factors:

FACTOR	FAVORABLE FACTOR	UNFAVORABLE
tumor size	small, less 1 cm	large tumor, 3cm
lymph nodes	no metastasis	metastasis
lymphatic intratumor invasion	absent	present
tumor differentiation	low grade 1 to 2	high grade 3 to 4
hormonal receptor	high	low
tumor growth rate s phase fraction	low	high
amount of DNA in cancer cell	diploid (normal)	aneuploid
Cathepsin D content	low	high
Her-2/neu expression	low	high
growth factors peptides	low	high

Q. What is the approximate survival with lymph node metastasis?

A. The following are approximate numbers:

Number of nodes	years after surgery	% survival
zero	2 years	98%
zero	5 years	90%
one	2 years	93%
one	5 years	80%
two - three	2 years	90%
two - three	5 years	75%
four - five	2 years	88%
four - five	5 years	68%
sixteen to twenty	2 years	75%
sixteen to twenty	5 years	48%

Q. How does the size of the tumor in the breast relate to probability of spread to the lymph nodes?

A. The larger the breast tumor, the greater the chance of spread to the lymph nodes.

Approximate spread to axillary lymph nodes:

Tumor size (2.5 cm = 1 inch)	*% of patients with nodal involvement*
less 0.5 cm	*20%*
0.5 to 0.9 cm	*20%*
1.5 to 1.9cm	*33%*
2.0 to 2.9 cm	*45%*
4.0 to 4.9 cm	*60%*
5.0 and greater	*70%*

Q. **What is a bone marrow transplant for breast cancer?**

A. For women that have a poorer prognosis, with greater than 10 nodes positive with cancer, some oncologists have suggested that the patient receive very high-dose chemotherapy in an attempt to kill any remaining cancer cells in the body. After the woman completes her normal chemotherapy, she has some of her bone marrow (where blood is made) removed and frozen so the bone marrow cells can be given back to her after she receives the very high-dose chemotherapy. Once the high-dose chemotherapy is given, it kills all the bone marrow cells. The patient must then spend about three to five weeks in the hospital after her frozen bone marrow cells are given back to her. During this time, she is at increased risk of infection because her blood count is very low. This treatment is not without risk and costs over one hundred thousand dollars. Some insurance companies will not pay for this treatment because how helpful the bone marrow transplant is in increasing survival is debated.

Q. **Can I return to work when receiving chemotherapy?**

A. Some women are able to work when undergoing treatment. This varies depending on the person.

Q. **Should I start an exercise problem when receiving chemotherapy?**

A. Only an established exercise program should be continued. Starting a new program, especially a vigorous one, may be too tiring.

Q. **I have heard that a special cap can be worn that prevents one's hair from falling out. Is this true?**

A. A special cap that cooled the scalp used to be used, but it has been found to be ineffective.

Q. **Do I need to avoid contact with people when I undergo chemotherapy?**

A. Usually one does not have to avoid any people unless the white blood count goes below 1000, which makes the patient susceptible to infection. This drop in the blood count occurs in about 50 percent of patients and is not permanent.

Q. **Do I need to have a special diet while receiving chemotherapy?**

A. It is not unusual for patients on chemotherapy to lose their appetites for awhile, so eating a well-balanced diet is suggested. A low-fat diet is recommended because it is often easier to digest. If your appetite is suppressed, you may want to add a multiple vitamin pill to ensure proper nutrition.

Q. **If I take extra vitamins, especially the antioxidants, will I have less chance of a recurrence of breast cancer?**

A. There is no conclusive evidence that taking antioxidants, such as vitamins C, E, and beta carotene, will improve a prognosis.

Q. **I've heard that taking chemotherapy will bring on menopause. Is that true?**

A. Most women over age 40 will go into permanent menopause. About 40 percent of women between ages 35 to 40 and about 25 percent of women between ages 30 to 35 will go into menopause after chemotherapy.

Q. **I have had no recurrence of my breast cancer for 5 years. Can I take estrogen for my bones to prevent osteoporosis?**

A. The correct answer to this question is not known. Most physicians feel estrogen does not cause cancer but that it may stimulate its growth. Because of possible lawsuits, claiming that estrogen causes cancer to recur, physicians are very cautious about recommending estrogens after a woman has breast cancer. Studies addressing this matter are currently in progress, but we will have to wait to see if the women taking estrogen develop recurrent cancer more frequently.

Q. **If my cancer does recur, when is it likely to happen?**

A. About 60 percent of all recurrent cancers occur in the first two years after treatment, and about 80 percent to 90 percent occur within five years of treatment. Only about 5 percent of recurrences occur within ten years after treatment.

Q. **What is the most important thing to do to catch any recurrence of cancer early?**

A. Approximately 90 percent of all recurrences are associated with some symptoms to the body, so it is a good idea to tell your physician of any new problems you have when you go for your routine check-ups. Physicians differ as to what tests, if any, need to be routinely performed in following a woman after she has received cancer treatment. With the trend to spend less healthcare dollars, physicians and patients will need to pay careful attention to any new health symptoms that arise.

Q. **Nurses have a difficult time placing IVs in my veins. Since chemotherapy must be given intravenously, how will I be able to receive treatment?**

A. There are two alternative ways for administering chemotherapy safely and easily if using arm veins is difficult. Both ways involve placing a long plastic catheter into one of the large veins (subclavian vein) that lies just below the collar bone. Placement is done by a surgeon as an outpatient surgical procedure.

Two catheters are available; the first is called an infus-a-port. The port is a small rubber reservoir that is placed under the skin and attaches to the long catheter that enters the vein. The main advantage of the infus-a-port is that the device is not visible, no home maintenance is required, and showering and swimming is not restricted. The disadvantage is that the skin must be punctured with a small needle to gain access to the vein.

The second catheter is also placed into the large subclavian vein, but the end of the catheter exits from the chest wall. The advantage with this catheter is that skin does not to be need to be punctured. However, since the tubing is exposed to air, special care is needed to keep the surrounding skin sterile and to prevent infection.

Chapter Eleven

PLASTIC SURGERY/ RECONSTRUCTION

(Bryan H. Pruitt, M.D.)

Q. What are the most important factors a woman should consider when selecting a plastic surgeon?

A. First, the surgeon should be eligible, or certified, by the American Board of Plastic Surgery, the only board for plastic surgeons recognized by the AMA and the American Board of Medical Specialties. Although some states are beginning to pass laws against them, several groups have created what are known as "bogus boards," with the words "plastic surgery" or "cosmetic surgery" in the name. They do not require the same extensive training and testing, and they are *not* recognized by the primary groups that certify doctors.

Second, when considering plastic surgery of the breast, a patient or her breast surgeon should seek out a plastic surgeon who has a great deal of experience in this special area and is able to offer the patient all possible options. Ask to see photographs of patients who will allow their photos to be used for patient education and find out if there are patients in the practice who have undergone the procedure who will talk with you.

Third, since plastic surgery of the breast is seldom done on an emergency basis, the patient should not hesitate to consult with more than one plastic surgeon if necessary until she finds one who best meets her needs and with whom she feels comfortable.

Q. **If I have breast reconstruction on my mastectomy site, will I need to have surgery on my other breast?**

A. Not necessarily. Most women do not require surgery on their remaining breast after a mastectomy. Some women, however, elect to do so in order to obtain a more symmetric result. Sometimes a breast lift or reduction surgery is performed so that the remaining breast will match the size of the reconstructed breast. Other women require augmentation of their normal breast so that it will not droop and will match the reconstructed breast more closely. And some women prefer to have a mastectomy of their remaining breast, a process used to virtually eliminate the risk of cancer developing in that breast. This way both breasts can be reconstructed simultaneously.

Q. **If my nipple is removed as a result of surgery, can the plastic surgeon reconstruct a new nipple, and where is he going to obtain the skin to do so?**

A. Yes, a nipple can be reconstructed using a new procedure that simply shapes the skin and tattoos it to make it look like a nipple. Previous older procedures involved removing skin from the groin, other breast nipple, skin from the upper thigh, tissue from the vulva, or from the ear lobe.

Q. **I understand that in some breast reconstruction cases, the plastic surgeon may recommend a tissue expander. Exactly what is this procedure?**

A. Before a plastic surgeon can place an implant, there first has to be enough skin and tissue available that can be stretched to accept a prothesis. The tissue is stretched very slowly, and to achieve this, a balloon filled with a saline solution is inserted under the pectoralis muscle. Every week or two, the surgeon injects additional saline, expanding the balloon. When the balloon has reached its desired size, it is removed and a prosthesis is inserted.

Tissue expanders can work very well in some patients and reduce the risks associated with placing an implant at the time of the mastectomy. The primary disadvantages of the tissue expanders are infection or erosion of the device through the skin. All of the risks associated with implant placement, such as capsular contracture or hardness, leakage, rupture, etc., are also a consideration.

Q. **I have heard on several television talk shows that implants can cause women to develop scleroderma and arthritis. Should I be concerned about this?**

A. There have been reports of arthritis or scleroderma occurring *after* implants. However, The American Rheumatology Association has suggested that implants not be placed in a woman if she has a history of autoimmune disease.

It has been rather difficult to establish any connection between implants and arthritis or scleroderma. Bear in mind that approximately 100,000 women in the United States have an implant each year. At the same time, approximately 30,000 women develop rheumatoid arthritis. Both implants and arthritis are very common. Consequently, women with or without implants may or may not develop arthritis or other medical problems. Research is going on in this area, but to date no conclusive cause and effect relationships have been identified. The *New England Journal of Medicine,* June 1994, reported that there is *no* association between connective tissue diseases such as lupus or rheumatoid arthritis and breast implants.

Q. **Can implants break, burst, or leak?**

A. Yes, it is now known that in the case of silicone-gel-filled breast implants, varying amounts of the silicone gel or liquid can leak out of the devices over time, a phenomena known as "gel bleed." The significance of the slow leakage is not known. This is not a problem with the implants that are filled with saline because, although they too can leak, the salt water or saline is readily absorbed.

Like all devices implanted in the body, breast implants

have some finite life span and can leak, crack, or rupture over time. It is important to remember that quite often an implant rupture is silent, meaning that neither the patient nor the doctor notices any problem, and the rupture is noted only on routine mammogram or at the time of implant exchange.

Q. **I have a friend who required the moving of a flap of skin to her chest wall after a mastectomy. Will I need the same reconstruction procedure for my breast when I have a mastectomy?**

A. Flaps are absolutely required in only a small number of reconstructions. They are utilized if: 1) the skin is too tight or thin following a mastectomy; 2) the pectoralis major muscle is absent or the nerves leading to the muscle cause the muscle to not function; 3) if a skin graft was used to close the chest wall; and, 4) if there is radiation damage to the chest wall following the mastectomy. There are, however, certain advantages to flap reconstruction that every patient should consider.

Q. **I had a subcutaneous mastectomy with implants performed because I had very lumpy breasts and my mother developed breast cancer. Do I still need to have regular mammograms?**

A. Definitely. Although you had a subcutaneous mastectomy, all the breast tissue was not removed. You can still develop a breast cancer. It is important for you to continue to perform breast self-exams *and* have mammograms!

Q. **In the reconstruction of breasts, there are several types of musculocutaneous flaps available. How do I know which type of flap is best?**

A. There are three main types of flaps used in breast reconstruction: Latissimus dorsi musculocutaneous, TRAM (transverse rectus abdominous musculocutaneous), and microvascular tram.

Each flap has very distinct advantages and disadvantages. The recommendation of a plastic surgeon on which one to use is based on each individual's anatomy and the amount of tissue transfer required.

The latissimus dorsi flap is the easiest to perform and many consider it to be the most dependable, but it usually requires an implant.

The TRAM flap probably provides the best cosmetic result, but it is a more difficult and prolonged procedure.

The microvascular TRAM flap is the new, high-tech way to do the TRAM in which the tissue is completely removed and attached to the blood vessels using microsurgical techniques. If a woman is to have this type flap, it is very important for the surgeon to have experience with this procedure and ensure the microsurgical techniques would work and that the correct vessels are present in the tissues preoperatively to perform this technique. ***(See Diagram, p. 132, 133)***

Q. **What is the scar tissue that develops around an implant?**

A. When any foreign body is implanted, the body's response is to wall off the object with scar, or fibrous, tissue. This scar formation is normal and helpful since it anchors the implant. If the scar tissue squeezes down around the implant, over time hardening and pain can result.

Q. **Is there a higher incidence of breast cancer in women who have had implants?**

A. There is no conclusive data that indicate that breast cancer is higher in women with implants. One of the largest studies of this subject involved over 3,000 women in Los Angeles County who were followed after implants. They showed no greater incidence of breast cancer.

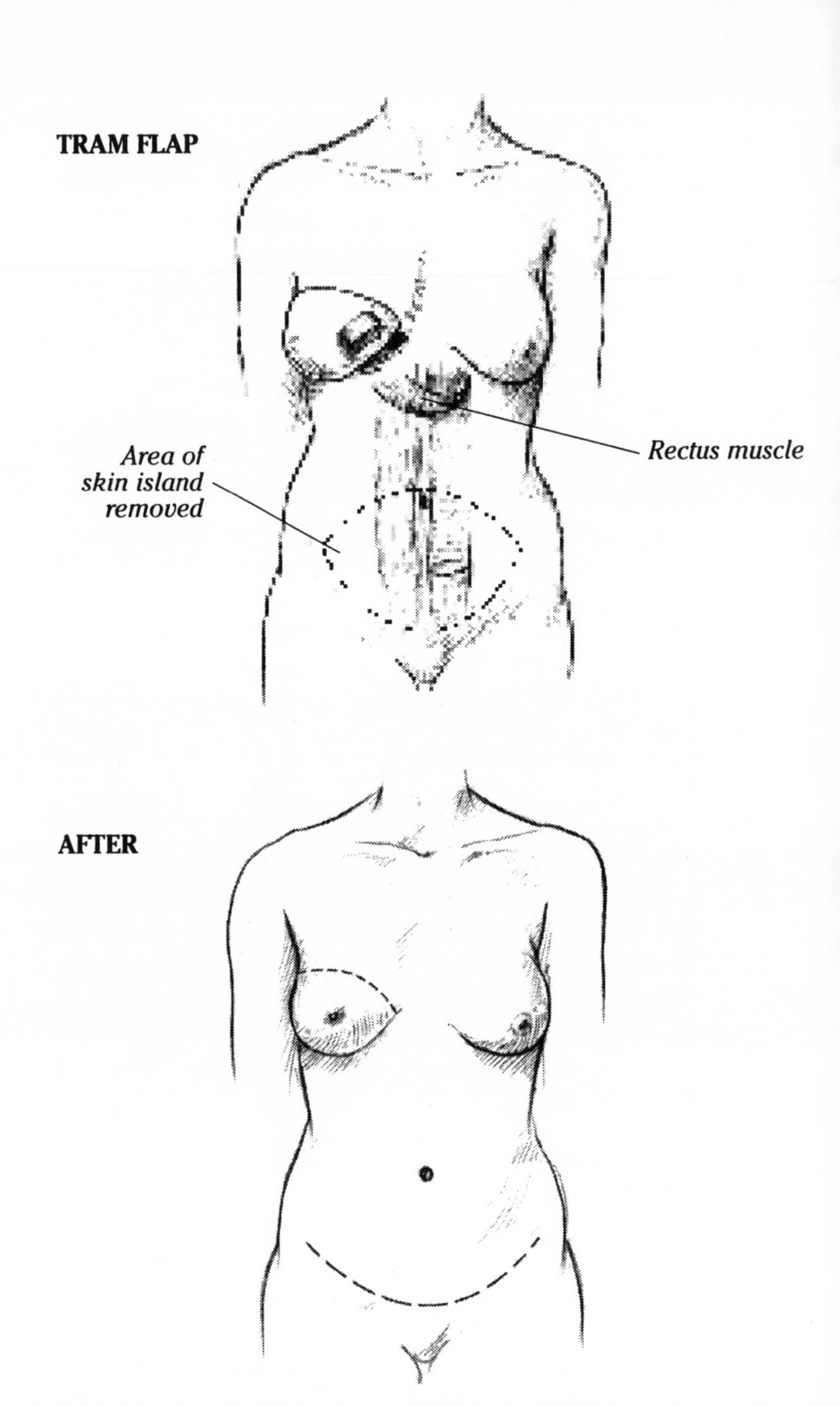
TRAM FLAP
Area of
skin island
removed
Rectus muscle
AFTER

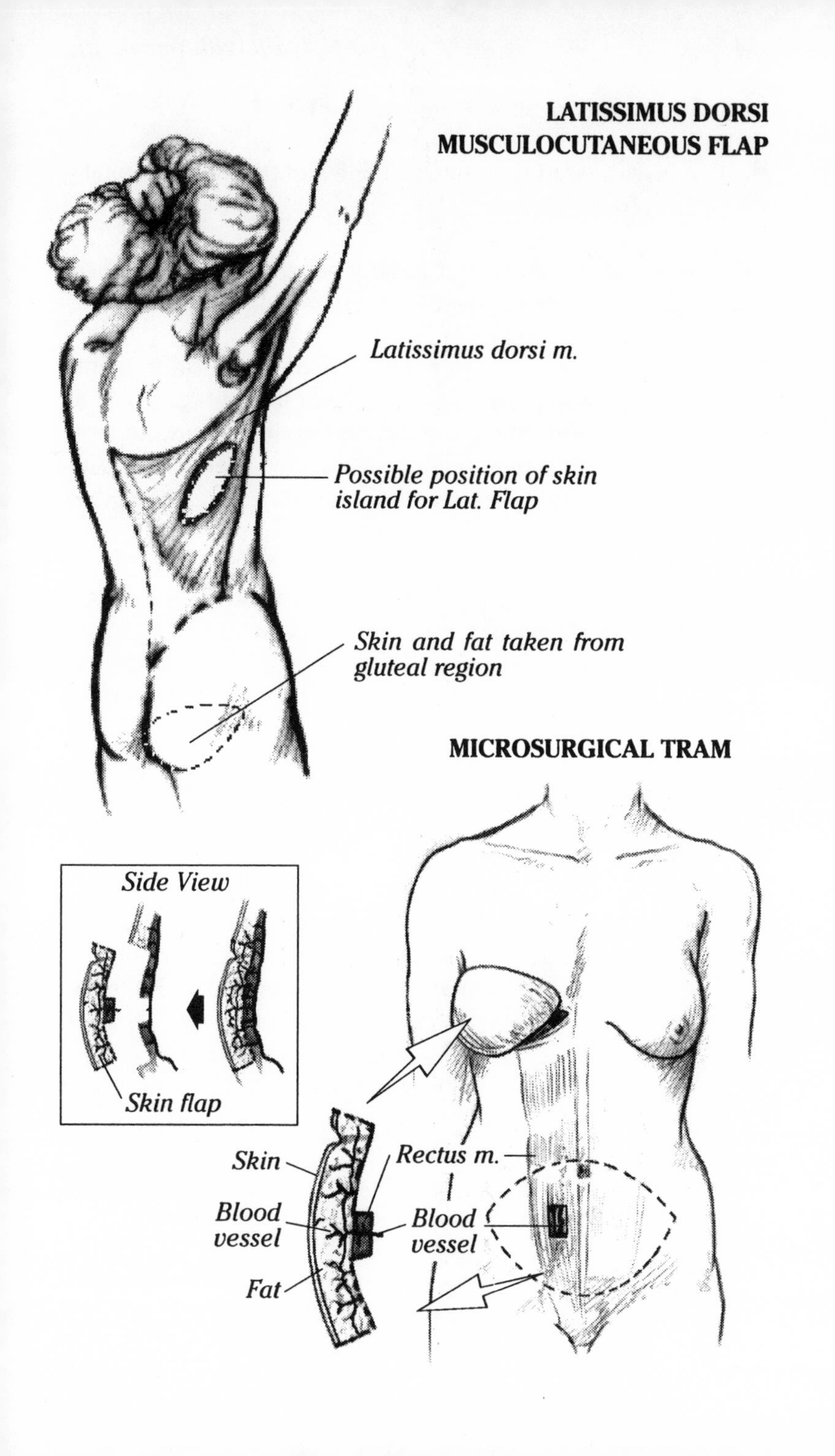
LATISSIMUS DORSI
MUSCULOCUTANEOUS FLAP
Latissimus dorsi m.
Possible position of skin
island for Lat. Flap
Skin and fat taken from
gluteal region
MICROSURGICAL TRAM
Side View
Skin flap
Skin
Blood
vessel
Fat
Rectus m.
Blood
vessel

Q. How many women have had implants?

A. It is estimated that between one and two million women have had implants.

Q. What is my chance of having severe scar tissue form after an implant, causing me to have hard breasts?

A. The risk is probably dependent on how long the implants have been in place, since a certain percentage per year become hard. The exact number varies widely, depending upon the type of implant, where they were placed anatomically, and how long they have been in place. Figures from 5 percent to 50 percent have been reported.

Q. What type of implant causes the least incidence of capsular scar formation and hard breasts?

A. Implants covered with polyurethane foam (which are no longer available) have the lowest rate of scar formation.

Q. What type of implant was taken off the market and for what reasons?

A. Polyurethane-covered implants have been voluntarily removed by the manufacturers. The implants have been removed because the body slowly breaks down polyurethane to 2,4-diaminotoluene, a substance which has caused liver cancer in experimental laboratory animals. The FDA does not recommend the removal of any intact implants that are not causing symptoms, since the risk of repeat surgery is felt to be greater than the theoretical risk of leaving the implants in place.

Q. Is there any alternative to silicone implants?

A. Saline-filled implants are available. This is like a balloon made of silicone which is filled with salt-water (saline).

One does not have to worry about silicone leakage since only salt-water can leak from the implant. The leakage rate is thought to be about 1 percent to 3 percent per year with the present models.

Q. Can implants be put in any special locations that will decrease the chance of a hard scar forming?

A. Implants placed beneath the pectoral muscle have been reported to have 50 percent less scar formation than implants placed above the muscle and in back of the breast tissue.

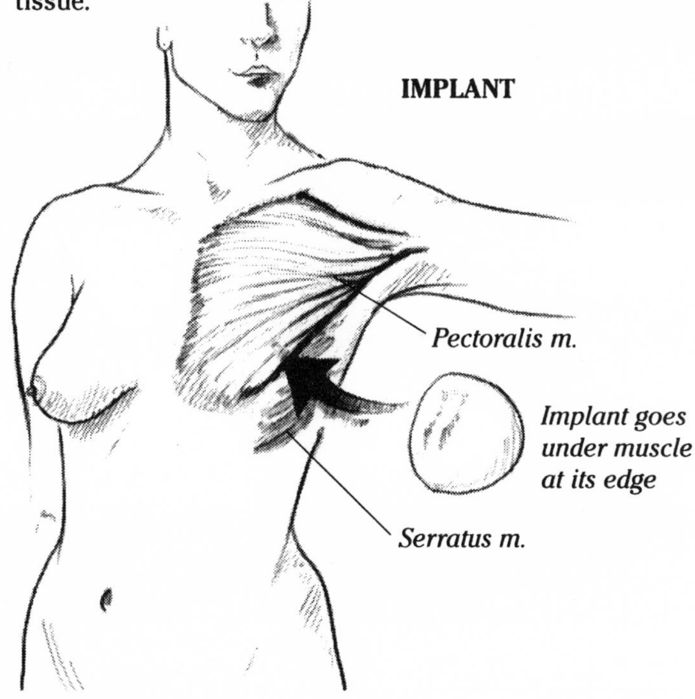

Q. Where is the incision made to insert an implant for breast enlargement?

A. The incision to insert the implant can be made in several places including: 1) under the breast; 2) in the armpit; or 3) around the areola (nipple).

Q. **Of what materials is an implant composed?**

A. Every implant has a solid silicone shell or bag. This shell is then filled with silicone gel, saline (salt water), or a mixture of saline and silicone.

Q. **I have heard that some of the newer implants have a different shell so there is less scar formation. How have they changed the shells?**

A. The outside shell of the implants have a textured surface so the implants have a rough surface. The textures cause the scar tissue to be irregular so the scar is softer.

The other technique has been to cover the implant with polyurethane; however, polyurethane implants have been voluntarily removed from the markets by the manufactures for theoretical health reasons.

Q. **At what age is it appropriate for a woman to consider breast augmentation (implants) or breast reduction?**

A. This is a very personal question and the answer varies with each individual. With the exception of gross asymmetry or deformity, breast augmentation surgery should not be considered until well after breast development has been complete. Since the decision to have breast implants placed can have such long-reaching effects, the older, more mature the girl, the better able she is to make an informed choice. Breast reduction may be necessary or desirable as early as the teenage years in some patients with abnormally large breasts.

Q. **If a woman is thinking about having plastic surgery on her breasts for cosmetic reasons only, would you recommend she have some psychological counseling first?**

A. In most cases, no. The desire to improve one's appearance is very natural and healthy. Psychologists have said that the desire to consider cosmetic surgery to enhance one's appearance is just as normal as the use of make-up, jewelry, hairstyling, or beautiful clothing. All of these can be part of a normal desire to look one's best. The most common, purely cosmetic, procedures of the breast include augmentation mammoplasty (breast enlargement with implants) and mastopexy or "breast lift."

Contrary to popular belief, most women who seek breast augmentation merely want an average, or normal, breast size, not abnormally large breasts or breasts out of proportion to their overall body size. Many are women in their thirties or forties who have already had children, have always wanted a more average breast size, and are considering the procedures for themselves, not out of a need for someone else's approval. After placement of breast implants, many women say that they have a wider choice of clothing options, an enhanced body image, and improved self esteem.

Mastopexy or "breast lift" is most often performed for women with sagging or drooping breasts that resulted from pregnancy, weight changes, or simply the effects of gravity over time (a part of aging).

Q. **What criteria is used to determine if plastic surgery on the breast is cosmetic or reconstructive surgery?**

A. This question can be answered by gaining an understanding of the differences between the two types of surgeries, as defined by the American Society of Plastic and Reconstructive Surgeons and the AMA:

Reconstructive surgery is surgery that is performed on abnormal structures of the body caused by congenital defects, developmental abnormalities, trauma, infection, tumors, or disease. It is generally performed to improve function but may also be done to approximate a normal appearance.

Cosmetic (aesthetic) surgery is defined as surgery to reshape normal structures of the body to improve the patient's appearance.

All of the surgery and other treatments provided by the plastic surgery specialty can be divided into one of these two categories. Sometimes two parts of one longer operation can fall separately into these two distinct categories.

(Note: Plastic surgeons and all other groups agree that cosmetic (aesthetic surgery) should not be covered by insurance or other health plans.)

Q. **Apart from cosmetic reasons or reconstruction after a mastectomy, for what other reasons would a woman need plastic surgery on her breasts?**

A. Many other plastic surgical procedures of the breasts are routinely performed. The most common is breast reduction surgery for excessively large, heavy breasts. Other conditions for which one might seek plastic surgical correction include congenital deformities, such as one breast that does not develop normally or that is very different in shape or size from the opposite breast, inverted nipples, contour deformities after lumpectomy and radiation, corrective surgery for those who have had implants placed and have experienced hardening or other problems, and many other conditions.

Q. **Does a typical health insurance policy cover any type of plastic surgery on breasts?**

A. Yes, all good health insurance policies cover any plastic surgical procedures considered to be reconstructive, but not those that are cosmetic in nature. (See definition above.) Most insurance companies will not pay for placement of breast implants (unless the patient has had some form of mastectomy or congenital deformity), or for "breast lifts" performed only to give the patient an improved, more youthful breast appearance. Virtually all other surgical procedures fall into the realm of reconstructive surgery and are routinely covered.

Q. **If, as a forty-three-year-old woman, I have my breasts enlarged with implants, will the implants need to be replaced in the future, say, when I am sixty or seventy?**

A. Breast implants, like all other devices, have some finite life span and over a long enough period of time may need to be replaced. The same is true for heart valves and most other devices implanted in the body. Technology continues to improve, however, and it is believed that the current devices are stronger and are likely to last longer than older models, but accurate long-term data on the devices currently used are not available.

Q. **If I have extremely large breasts, are there any physiological benefits to having them surgically reduced?**

A. Yes. Breast reduction surgery is almost always performed to alleviate symptoms involving shoulder pain, severe bra strap grooving of the shoulders, neck and back pain resulting from carrying such a heavy weight in this forward position, and skin disorders or rashes from the dark, moist, skin-to-skin contact beneath the breasts. Studies show that these symptoms are greatly improved or relieved in most patients.

Q. **Would you discuss the silicone gel controversy?**

A. Since 1963, between one and two million women have undergone placement of silicone devices, both for breast reconstruction after mastectomy and for breast augmentation, or enlargement. When these devices are implanted, the body forms a "capsule" of fibrous tissue around them. In some patients, too much of this tissue forms, leading to the most common long and short term problem after surgery: breasts that are too hard, misshapen, or even painful. In some studies, capsular contracture, as this problem is called, has been reported to occur in up to 50 percent of breast implant patients, although most do not consider it severe enough to seek surgical correction. New surgical techniques and improved implant designs appear to be decreasing this problem. Other risks which are much less common are also known to occur in extremely small percentages of patients and are always discussed with patients considering this type of surgery.

The controversy has centered on the following questions:

Do breast implants cause cancer? No reliable scientific or medical evidence has proven this to be true. Although certain rodents have been shown to form a different type of neoplasms with silicone implants in place, studies of large groups of women with implants reveal that they are no more likely to develop breast cancer than other women. A recent study reported from Canada further documents that women with breast implants who develop breast cancer had no statistical difference in long-term survival compared with those who did not have breast implants. Because such a large number of women have breast implants and because the incidence of breast cancer in this country is so high and climbing (one in every nine women) there will certainly continue to be women with breast implants in place who will develop cancer. This does not mean that the implants *caused* the cancer, but merely that both are present in the same patient.

Do implants interfere with mammography? Breast implants, both saline and silicone, can reduce the amount of breast tissue clearly visualized on mammography. Even with the special additional views that are routinely performed on patients with implants by experienced centers, a portion of the breast tissue may not be adequately imaged. Although most studies of breast implant patients who go on to develop breast cancer show no difference in the stage at presentation or the long-term cure rates, all patients considering breast implants should understand that, even in the best mammography centers, implants may limit to some degree the percentage of breast tissue that can be reliably imaged.

Does the silicone gel or liquid silicone come out of the implants or go to other parts of the body? Yes. Recent studies have confirmed that some silicone gel comes out through the shell and into the surrounding tissue, even in implants that are not ruptured. In patients with silicone gel implants, silicone has been identified in the breast capsule, breast tissue, lymph nodes, and even some distant sites in the body, such as the liver and spleen (although the amounts in these distant sites is difficult to measure and may be no greater than that of the population at large). The significance of this "migration," if any, is currently unknown.

Does silicone gel cause any generalized or systemic disease, including those associated with the immune system? Some women with breast implants and their doctors have expressed concern about symptoms including chronic fatigue, arthritis or joint pain and swelling, skin rashes, and a variety of other symptoms. Research is in progress in these areas, but so far no scientific cause and effect have been demonstrated. A June 1994 study from the Mayo Clinic concluded that there is *no* association between implants and the connective tissue diseases, including rheumatoid arthritis, lupus, and many other conditions.

Q. **If a patient needing reconstruction didn't want silicone gel implants, would she have other options?**

A. Yes, a multitude of options are available, some using only the patient's own tissue.

Q. Tissue transplantation, taking tissue from another fatty part of the body like the tummy or the buttocks, would seem to me to be an ideal option, yet this is rather uncommon. Why?

A. It *is* an ideal option for many patients, and it is becoming more and more common every year. But understand, these kinds of surgery are relatively new, high-tech operations, requiring the transfer of tissue, sometimes using the operating microscope to make microvascular anastomosis (joining) of vessels. Most plastic surgeons have little experience with these types of breast reconstructions. As more surgeons acquire the skills to perform these procedures, and as the benefits of using the patient's own tissue become more widely known, this type of breast reconstruction will no doubt increase, unless government or "managed care" force surgeons to continue with more "cost-effective" (cheaper) methods.

Q. How much pain is associated with a "simple" breast reduction? A simple breast enlargement?

A. The amount of pain or discomfort associated with either breast reduction or breast enlargement varies with the individual patients. Most patients require only oral pain pills after surgery.

Q. What kind of recovery period should a healthy patient expect if she has had breast augmentation? Breast reduction surgery?

A. Depending on the woman's usual daily activities or type of work, most women can return to their routine within a few days after either type of procedure. Most surgeons would prohibit heavy physical activity or exertion for several days to two weeks, especially overhead lifting. If sutures have to be removed, this will be done in the surgeon's office a few days after the surgery. Slight swelling or bruising will subside over a few weeks, and the patient's breasts should then be their final size.

Q. **How soon can reconstructive surgery be performed on a mastectomy patient?**

A. Reconstruction can begin immediately after completion of the mastectomy, during the same anesthesia.

Q. **What exactly is "immediate reconstruction," and under what circumstances would you recommend it?**

A. Immediate reconstruction refers to this relatively new concept of proceeding with reconstruction at the time of the mastectomy, so the woman never has to go for a period of time without a breast mound.

It was formerly thought that early or immediate reconstruction might delay the detection of a recurrence of the breast cancer or interfere with subsequent therapy. And since a reconstructed breast seldom, if ever, looks *exactly* like the natural breast, it was felt that the patient could not appreciate the reconstruction until she had experienced the mastectomy defect for some period of time. Several studies have proven both of these concerns to be invalid. A reconstructed breast is at no greater risk of recurrent cancer, and patients indicate a much higher level of satisfaction with only a single anesthetic, a single recovery period, and a significant overall reduction in costs.

With few exceptions, most women are candidates for immediate breast reconstruction at the time of their mastectomy.

Q. **If I'm undergoing chemotherapy, is it necessary for me to delay reconstruction?**

A. No. This concern has been studied in centers where large numbers of breast cancer patients are treated and reconstruction is performed, and it was found to be very unusual for immediate reconstruction to cause any delay. Chemotherapy is routinely begun and continued on schedule in patients who choose immediate breast reconstruction.

Q. **What circumstances would cause you to recommend delaying reconstructive surgery?**

A. Breast reconstruction is generally delayed in 1) patients who will need radiation therapy to the breast region; 2) patients who have a concurrent infection or inflammation in the region; or, 3) patients who might have a serious current health problem, such as a recent heart attack. In a situation of this type, the patient's risks can be improved by minimizing the magnitude of the surgery and proceeding when the condition stabilizes.

Q. **Are most mastectomy patients viable candidates for reconstruction?**

A. Yes, almost all mastectomy patients are now considered to be candidates for breast reconstruction.

Q. **What circumstances would cause a plastic surgeon to discourage a patient from undergoing reconstruction?**

A. Only severe medical problems that would dramatically increase the risk of any type of surgery would absolutely preclude any breast reconstruction. Other more relative factors would depend more on the magnitude of the particular type of breast reconstruction being considered.

Q. **Are skin grafts always needed for reconstruction after a mastectomy?**

A. No. Additional tissue is often needed for the best reconstruction, but instead of skin grafts, this tissue is usually taken from the lower tummy, back, or buttocks.

Q. **What is the normal recovery period after reconstruction?**

A. The recovery period varies with the type of reconstruction chosen. It can range from a few days to a few weeks for complete healing and recovery.

Q. **During the mastectomy, are there some things the surgeon can do to prepare the way for reconstructive surgery?**

A. Absolutely. The plastic surgeon can achieve a much better overall result if during the mastectomy the breast surgeon has been careful to leave intact the fold under the breast and the nerves and blood vessels going to the chest wall muscles.

Q. **How important is a patient's age in considering reconstructive surgery?**

A. Although age is a factor to consider, the woman's overall health is more important. A woman is never too old to feel the desire to be "whole," and these procedures have been performed in patients whose chronological age is quite advanced.

Q. **What percentage of mastectomy patients choose to have reconstructive surgery?**

A. This varies widely among different regions of the country and even among different institutions within the same region or city. This variance is probably related more to the attitudes of the surgeons performing the mastectomies and the availability of a trained plastic surgeon than any other factors.

Q. **Does a woman with implants need special follow-up examinations, in addition to her annual exams and mammogram?**

A. Yes. Most physicians now recommend a yearly visit with a plastic surgeon to follow the implants and the patient's body's reaction to them.

Q. **How does a woman with implants do breast self-exams?**

A. These should be performed in the same way women without implants perform them. (See Chapter 3) Any mass, changes, irregularities, or nipple discharge should be reported to a breast surgeon or plastic surgeon as soon as possible.

Q. **Can anything be done to prevent breast implants from hardening?**

A. When any device is implanted within the body, a natural encapsulating occurs, which means that a scar membrane called a "capsule" forms around the device as the body heals. In the case of breast implants, if the scar capsule remains thin and pliable, the breast will continue to be soft and natural appearing. If, however, for reasons that are currently unknown, the capsule thickens, the firmness can increase, causing a condition that is called capsular contraction. Although a mild degree of firmness may be desirable for some women, if firmness continues to increase, the breasts can become misshapen, hard, and even painful. This abnormal encapsulation may occur immediately after surgery, or it may not occur until many years later, occurring on only one side or on both.

Research has been unable to prove any clear cause for capsular contraction, although some studies show rates of over 50 percent for this abnormal firmness in cases where older, smooth-walled devices were implanted. A great deal of active research is underway, and the most recent development indicates that a textured coating of the implants (instead of just a smoother shell) decreases the risk of this excessive firmness occurring. As a result, implants of this type are now being used regularly.

Research surveys of women with capsular contraction have shown that even in severe cases, most patients do not feel that it is bothersome enough to request removal of the devices. If severe capsular contracture does occur and the woman wishes to have this corrected, she can discuss with her plastic surgeon various methods of interrupting the scar tissue (capsulotomy) or removing it surgically (capsulectomy). Even when soft breasts are again achieved, the capsular contracture may recur.

Q. **If I have my breasts enlarged and later regret it, can the implants be safely removed?**

A. Yes. The appearance of the breasts may not be what they were prior to the breast enlargement because of the stretching of the tissue and aging, but the devices can be removed. In the case of silicone gel-filled implants, it is probably not possible to ever completely remove all traces of the liquid silicone, but the vast majority can be removed.

Q. **What are the advantages and disadvantages of breast reconstruction implants versus breast reconstruction using the patient's own fatty tissue?**

A. IMPLANTS

Advantages

—Initial operation simpler, easier to perform with less time in the hospital and fewer risks;

—More plastic surgeons have the training to perform this type of reconstruction;

—The option to remove the implants and use the patient's own tissue is usually still available.

Disadvantages

—May require two or three separate operations if expansion of the tissue is needed, followed by exchange of the

expander for an implant, and then nipple reconstruction;
—The breast implant is a device, and future concerns about hardness, leakage, replacement, etc., must be addressed;
—Multiple future procedures may increase total costs.

PATIENT'S OWN TISSUE

Advantages

—Once the reconstruction is completed, there is very little chance of ever needing any further surgery;
—Excellent appearance, shape, and contour;
—Enhancement of donor site, i.e., removal of "tummy tuck" tissue;
—Very high patient satisfaction.

Disadvantages

—Longer, more involved initial procedure;
—Longer hospital stay and post-operative recovery;
—Higher initial costs.

Q. **If I have already had breast reconstruction after a mastectomy or subcutaneous mastectomy with implants, and my implants leak, rupture, or get hard, do I have to have them replaced with *more* implants, or is the use of my "tummy tuck" tissue still an option?**

A. This is a very common question, asked by many women. In most cases, the answer is you do *not* have to have more implants placed; and if excess skin and fat are available on your tummy, buttocks, or elsewhere, this may be used for the reconstruction after the old implants are removed.

Q. **Are most women who choose to have breast implants placed for breast enlargement happy with the long term results?**

A. Yes, studies have shown that more than 90 percent of women surveyed who had had implants were happy with the results.

Q. **What is a breast lift or "uplifting procedure," and what women are candidates for this?**

A. Breast lifting, also known as "mastopexy," is performed to elevate the breast tissue and nipple, giving the overall breast appearance a more attractive, youthful, or aesthetically pleasing form.

The sagging or drooping (known clinically as "ptosis") can result from the hormonal and breast-size changes associated with pregnancy and breast-feeding, overall fluctuations in the patient's weight, or just the effects of gravity on the breasts over time (a component of aging). A variety of techniques can be employed to perform this "uplifting," with the newest techniques focusing on reducing incisions to a minimum. Breast lifting procedures can produce excellent improvement in overall shape and appearance.

Q. **Can anything be done to improve the sensation of a reconstructed breast?**

A. Yes, one of the very latest frontiers in breast reconstruction is microscopic nerve repair to improve sensation in the new breast.

Chapter Twelve

THE EMOTIONS OF BREAST CANCER

Q&A **Did I bring this cancer on myself?**

Cancer happens to all types of people. We know that your thoughts or actions are not the cause of your breast cancer. Recent research indicates that there is no specific "cancer personality" that might be the cause of cancer.

Q. **I have a lot of stress in my life. Is it possible that this is a cause of my breast cancer?**

A. Everyone has stress in life and people respond to the stress differently. And it is true that stress does have an adverse affect on the immune system, but we do not know how this relates to breast cancer, if at all.

Q. **I am angry that I developed breast cancer. Is this normal?**

A. Yes, anger is a normal response to the discovery that you have breast cancer. Women often experience anger towards God, their doctor, or even their breast once they have been told that they have breast cancer. Allow yourself to feel and express your anger. You can expect that it will decrease over time.

Q. **Do women who have a lumpectomy instead of a mastectomy have less psychological difficulties after treatment?**

A. There is no conclusive proof that women who have conservative treatment of a lumpectomy and radiation treatment do any better psychologically in the long run than women who have a mastectomy. It is my experience that many women are more concerned initially about their life expectancy and the recurrence of the cancer than with the loss of their breast. While the long term psychological adjustments are similar, a mastectomy can be psychologically traumatic. Many women experience this after their treatment. Individuals vary greatly in their emotional responses to the loss of a breast.

Q. **I feel like everyone is treating me as though cancer were a contagious disease. It isn't, is it?**

A. There is no evidence that breast cancer is contagious. Your friends and family need to understand this so that they can treat you normally. It would be a good idea for them to learn as much about the disease as possible—this will not only put them at ease with you but also will enable them to be a source of encouragement to you.

Q. **I am afraid that having breast cancer might harm my sexual relationship with my husband. Is this a normal fear? What can I do to rid myself of this fear?**

A. Yes, this is a normal fear. In our culture, women's breasts are associated with sexuality and attractiveness, whether we like it or not. So for many women who have had a mastectomy or a lumpectomy and radiation, the idea of a breast that is scarred or diseased carries with it added concerns and fears, beyond the health issue. As with most difficulties within marriage, the best solution is good communication. Most couples can work through the problems that occur as a natural by-product of change (almost any kind of cancer is a frightening change within a marriage) if they are willing to talk and listen to one another with honesty, patience, and understanding. If this kind of communication is difficult or impossible for you and your husband, a professional counselor can help you learn communication techniques that will be helpful in resolving any sexual and emotional problems that may have resulted from your breast cancer.

Q. **Where can I go for support after my breast cancer?**

A. Most areas have support groups for women who have breast cancer. These groups are comprised of women who have had breast cancer and who meet together to encourage one another and offer one another mutual support and information. Your surgeon or a hospital social worker should be able to refer you to a local group. In my opinion, one of the best resources for finding a support group in your area is an organization called Reach for Recovery. They should be listed in the Yellow Pages of your telephone book, or you can get information about them by calling the American Cancer Society (1-800-ACS-2345). Many groups have a professional facilitator who helps to direct breast cancer patients into support groups. For many women, having a support group to share their experience of breast cancer has been an important part of their recovery.

Q. **What is Reach for Recovery?**

A. Reach for Recovery is a volunteer organization made up of women who have had either a mastectomy or a lumpectomy with radiation treatment. They meet with breast cancer patients after surgery and bring them a pamphlet explaining the exercises they can do after surgery. They also bring a temporary prothesis a woman can wear right away and offer her help in obtaining a more permanent prothesis. Reach for Recovery volunteers can usually suggest local support groups where women can find help in working through the psychological aspects of having breast cancer.

Q. **Is there any evidence to suggest that a husband is more likely to leave his wife after she has been diagnosed with breast cancer?**

A. No. There is no conclusive evidence that would cause us to believe that men leave their wives any more frequently after breast cancer than they would if their wives had not developed breast cancer. If the marriage is healthy to begin with, a man who had not considered leaving his wife *before* her breast cancer is not likely to leave her *after* her diagnosis and treatment.

Q. **What are some ways that family and friends can help meet the emotional needs of the woman who has recently been diagnosed with breast cancer?**

A. The most helpful thing that family members and friends can do during this period is to accept the emotions that the patient is currently experiencing. By doing this they can provide a safe environment in which she can identify and express her feelings and thoughts, which is the first step towards coping with this emotionally difficult period. It is important to neither minimize the situation, nor make it into a catastrophe. Family and friends understandably want the patient to be free of painful emotions. They may at times try to persuade her to feel differently than she does, but this kind of persuasion rarely helps—we cannot force ourselves or anyone else to experience feelings on demand. It is helpful for the support persons, as well as the patient herself, to remember that feelings change; they are not permanent. Today's emotions may be very different tomorrow. Support for the newly diagnosed patient should also include fundamental information about the disease. She should be encouraged to avoid the terrifying "what ifs" and to keep her thoughts based in reality. It is also very important to convey a sense of hopefulness regarding the disease and to allow the individual the necessary time to grieve over this loss and the sudden change in her life.

During this time, support persons will also need to deal with their own feelings about their loved one's cancer diagnosis.

Q. **Is it true that physical recovery from breast cancer is sometimes easier than the psychological recovery?**

A. Many women report this to be true. The physical recovery from surgery for breast cancer is relatively short-term and uncomplicated for most women; the psychological adjustment to changes in their body image, adapting to the reality of having cancer and dealing with fears of recurrent disease is a long process. The surgery and the disease may cause past losses and experiences to resurface and complicate the process of recovery. Each check-up or ache may cause emotions to resurface and demand further attention. It is important to see the recovery process as ongoing, with no clearly delineated point of completion. This lack of a specific time frame can be extremely frustrating for women. Keep in mind, most women make an adaptive psychological recovery from the trauma of breast cancer and lead emotionally full and gratifying lives.

Q. **Is the patient's attitude an important factor when choices of cancer treatment are being considered?**

A. It is vital that the healthcare team consider the patient's attitude when forming the treatment plan. A woman's attitudes regarding the possible loss of her breast and her accompanying fears of disfigurement should be considered as a factor regarding surgical treatment of her breast cancer. A woman's experiences with other family or friends who have had breast cancer may affect her attitude and increase her anxiety regarding her chance of being cured. Fear of chemotherapy may well impact treatment plans. Generally, if the healthcare team is well aware of the patient's attitudes, they are able to develop a treatment plan that the patient can tolerate, which will also increase the likelihood of good patient co-operation.

Q. **Is there one best way to encourage hope and engender a positive attitude in a woman diagnosed with breast cancer?**

A. There is no single method which accomplishes this in all women who are coping with breast cancer. Individuals differ in what they find gives them a sense of hope and helps them to maintain a positive attitude. Information that is accurate and correctly understood is helpful for most women. This is especially true of information that stresses that they may impact the course of their disease to some degree. Focusing on their individual strengths and successes may help patients rally their own resources.

Contact with other breast cancer survivors can be of great benefit to newly diagnosed patients. It allows them to see that survival is possible and that life *can* return to normal, and that, in fact, life may even be enriched in some ways because of this experience.

Q. **What are some ways that patients can learn to manage their anxiety?**

A. Many cancer patients have found ways to manage the extremely uncomfortable but unavoidable emotion of anxiety that comes with their disease. Because feeling out of control is a common feeling of cancer patients, many women find that their anxiety is decreased when they increase their knowledge of the disease and when they become involved in treatment options. Learning all they can and taking control in areas in which it is feasible helps patients feel more in control of their lives and lessens feelings of anxiety. Taking control may involve major issues or small but emotionally significant ones, like the day of the week on which treatment is given. But regardless, every opportunity increases the patient's feelings of control.

In addition, when patients are allowed to openly discuss their fears and explore them realistically, they can discover strategies for adapting to their disease. Using available support, family and friends, healthcare providers, church, and support groups can also be healthy ways of handling feelings. They are often able to help reduce a patient's sense of isolation, decrease her anxiety, and help her make a positive adjustment to her disease.

Q. **What seems to help women get through chemotherapy and radiation?**

A. Neither chemotherapy nor radiation therapy is pleasant. Women experience a wide variety of side effects, in varying degrees. Going into treatment with a positive attitude will help you cope with whatever side effects you might encounter. A patient's fears regarding treatment can be reduced if she is assured that most symptoms can be well managed. Patients can help the physician better manage their care and help create a team approach to their treatment if they will communicate with their doctors about any problems or symptoms they have. *Never assume that nothing can be done*. Communicate problems in as specific a way as possible. Your doctor cannot know what you don't tell her.

It is important for you to be realistic regarding what you can and cannot do throughout the duration of your treatment and then, to be able to adapt to these limitations. Pushing yourself too hard will slow down your recovery and put an added stress on your body. So get adequate rest, accept help, and let things slide a little.

Keep your life as normal as possible. Distraction is a

wonderful coping strategy. Continuing to be involved in activities that are important to you reassures you that a substantial part of your life is still normal, which keeps you connected with the world. Women who stay interested and involved experience less depression, so use your mind to help you through this time. Remind yourself that treatment is temporary and that any problems you may experience are related to the treatment, not the disease. Remember, treatment is your best chance for a cure. In other words, try not to mentally fight the treatment. See it as an ally rather than an enemy.

Q. **I've survived breast cancer, but I can't seem to get rid of my fears that it will return. Can my fears and the stresses they produce contribute to the disease returning?**

A. First of all, it is important for you to know how normal these fears are. Almost all cancer patients experience fears that their disease may return—the fact that cancer *can* recur is one factor that makes it so frightening.

There is no proof that stress or fear causes the development of cancer in the first place, nor that it can cause a recurrence of the disease; however, these fears and the stresses they produce *do* affect your body and its immune system. This may be one factor that affects the path of your disease.

While we are not sure to what extent these stresses affect your disease, we do know that they significantly impact the quality of your life on a day-to-day basis. So, whether you have five months or fifty years to live, it is best to try to live without extreme fear. To do this, you will need to learn to manage your fears and stresses.

If you allow yourself to believe that you have somehow caused your disease, or that you can cause its recurrence, you will create added anxiety, as well as guilt; this can hinder your ability to manage your fears and adapt to your disease.

Q. **Treatment is finished, and my prognosis is good. Everyone seems to think it is all over and that I should feel great. However, I feel worse emotionally than before. Is this normal, or am I going crazy?**

A. This is a common situation, and it is confusing for both the patient and her support persons. There are several factors that may contribute to this. It takes a great deal of time and energy to deal with getting through treatment. Often there is little energy left over to process the emotional aspects of the disease, and emotions may take a back burner to the demands of treatment. When treatment is over, these suppressed emotions tend to break through, bringing with them a heightened awareness of what has happened to you and what you have been through. Like many other crises in our lives, we do what we must to get through, and then we allow ourselves to become emotional. As your treatment ends, for the first time you may become aware of how drastically the disease has changed your life and of the ways that your life will always be different. While there may be positive as well as negative changes, few would have chosen cancer as a way to change their lives.

Finally, there is the fact that you are no longer doing anything about the cancer. As much as most women want to be finished with treatment, many experience some anxiety about the safety of stopping treatment, and they worry about whether or not careful monitoring is enough. Treatment may have made them feel more secure.

The post-treatment period can be a very difficult time. Do not hesitate to get any help you may need.

Q. **I have young children. What should I tell them about my cancer?**

A. Regardless of your children's ages, you need to be honest and open with them regarding the diagnosis and treatment.

Using simple terms that are appropriate for their ages, explain what breast cancer is and what treatment you plan to receive. Emphasize that the treatment has some side effects, but that it is being done to cure the disease. Often, children gain a better sense of what is happening if you take them with you for treatments and allow them to meet your doctor. Do not avoid telling them that people can die of cancer—most children know this or will hear it some time. Instead, tell them that people can die of cancer, but you and your doctors are doing all you can to make you well. Reassure them that most women survive breast cancer; explain that you will not feel well for a while but that you will get back to being yourself. Also, it is important to be reminded that children often blame themselves for things. Assure them that nothing they said or did or thought caused you to become ill.

Remember, children pick up on their parents' emotional states—they always know when something is wrong. If you try to conceal facts, children will try their best to make sense of the emotional situation in which they find themselves. This is unfair to a child. Like adults, information allows children to cope better.

Q. **How can I expect the surgery to affect my sexuality?**

A. Most women have serious concerns regarding their sexuality after surgery. Some women are unsure of how their husband will feel about them after surgery. They may fear rejection. It is important to know that most women return to a satisfying sexual life after surgery for breast cancer. Do not avoid discussing your fears and concerns with your partner. Accept that it may take time for the two of you to adjust to this change. For most women it helps to resume sexual activity as soon as you feel physically able. This is a time when you both very much need the emotional closeness that most couples experience through sexual relations. It also helps to have the reassurance that this part of your lives is still there for you. If problems develop and persist over time, get professional help to work through them. Problems are not inevitable, and often, relationship problems that are surfacing at this time are not solely a result of breast cancer. If your relationship is a good one and your sexual life has been gratifying, this experience should not damage that. In fact, many find that after the diagnosis their relationship grows even deeper. They are more aware of how important they are to one another, and they are more appreciative of the time they have together.

Q. **As a single woman, I worry about how to handle dating and relationships.**

A. It is very difficult for single women to think about dating and forming a relationship after surgery. Questions about how and when to talk about this part of your life are understandable. There are no clear and absolute answers. Honesty is an important part of all healthy relationships and the fact of having had breast cancer is no exception. There is no reason that anyone should avoid having a full and normal life after breast cancer. If dating and sexuality are an important part of that for you, it can continue to be a part of life. Keep in mind that many factors go into sexual attraction and satisfaction.

Q. **Is it important psychologically to have breast reconstruction done?**

A. Breast reconstruction is a wonderful option for many women; however, it is a very individual choice. Some women are comforted by the fact that they will have reconstruction surgery. This may help them to better cope with surgery and treatment. Many women express the feeling that reconstructive surgery allows them to put the cancer experience behind them and move on without the visual reminders of what they have been through. Other women make the choice because they find a prosthesis uncomfortable. Finally, some women do not feel the need for reconstructive surgery. This may mean they are satisfied with their appearance. For some, it reflects the desire to have no further medical procedures. Keep in mind this is an individual choice. A woman should have reconstructive surgery because she wants it and understands what it will and will not do for her. One is not too old to care about such things, nor is it an indication of being vain. It can be a healthy manifestation of coping, but it is not essential for good psychological adjustment. (Note: As of this writing, the Clinton administration's proposed healthcare plan would not pay for any breast reconstruction.)

Q. **I am very concerned about how my cancer is affecting my family. What can I do to help them?**

A. Cancer does not happen to individuals; it happens to families. It is inevitable that your having cancer will have a significant impact on your family. Women often feel guilty when they see their family distressed about their disease. Some express guilt about "what they are doing to their family." But *you* are not doing this to your family, *cancer* is affecting you and your family. Each member of your family needs to express whatever feelings they may have about your illness. This can include anger that you are unable to do things you usually do for them, fear that they might lose you, worries about treatment, guilt, or sadness. Give your family members a chance to talk with you and others about what is happening to the family. Try and keep life as normal as possible for each family member. Offer reassurance and hope to those who care about you. Let your family help you. Nothing makes you feel as helpless as having nothing to do when someone you love is going through a difficult time. Finally, remember that this is a difficult time for all of you. You will all survive. As much as we would like to protect those we love from anything painful, we cannot. Families can grow and become stronger as a result of this experience.

Q. **What are the most common emotional responses you see in patients recently diagnosed with breast cancer?**

A. While individuals may vary greatly in the type and degree of emotions they experience, some of the most common responses include anxiety, sadness, fear, disbelief, a sense of numbness, a feeling of unreality or disconnection, feelings of being overwhelmed, anger, guilt, fear of abandonment, frustration, and helplessness. They may also experience a sense of confusion, distractibility, irritability, and disorientation. Not all individuals experience all these emotions, nor is it necessary for them to do so. What specific emotions the individual experiences, the degree of the emotional distress, and how this distress is manifested depends on the personality of the individual. We each have our own personality structure and our own distinct ways of experiencing and responding to the events of our lives. This personality, formed in part by the sum of past experiences, is the most important factor in determining what an individual may experience or how they may react to the experiences they encounter. However, most breast cancer patients will experience a significant number of the above emotions at various times, especially at the time of the diagnosis.

Q. **How might these feelings manifest themselves?**

A. Common manifestations would include tearfulness, emotional lability (the sudden onset or shift of emotional states), difficulty focusing and concentrating, anger outbursts, agitation (difficulty being still), and distractibility. Some patients may appear devoid of emotions, reacting in an extremely matter-of-fact way, very concerned with practical issues. Some patients may be completely preoccupied with the diagnosis, while others may act as though nothing has happened and focus on other things. It is important to note that these are all normal manifestations of understandable and normal feelings. They represent the patients' attempts to adapt to an emotionally painful and threatening situation. If there is little or no change over time, or if the manifestations of their emotions interfere with their treatment, intervention is necessary. For most, this is not the case; they achieve a balanced and tolerable emotional state that allows them to function in a healthy and rational way. If you find yourself at any time struggling with coping with your feelings, do not hesitate to get professional help. Do not try to struggle through on your own. The whole point is to make a healthy recovery.

A MESSAGE FROM THE PUBLISHER

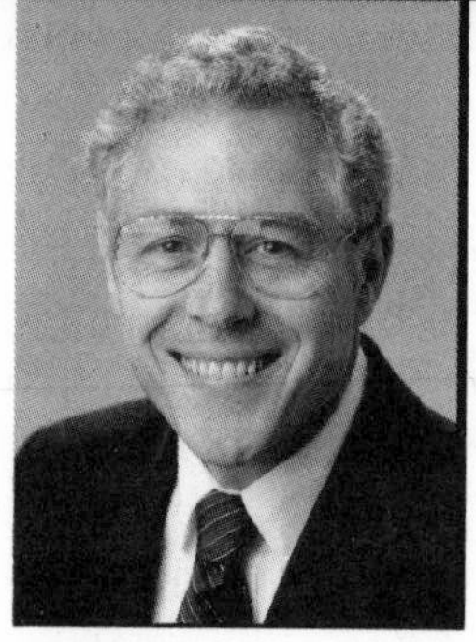

W. R. Spence, M.D.
Publisher

In 1975 I made the first commercially available breast cancer teaching model. It found little professional or public interest until Betty Ford's highly publicized cancer. Since that time our health education company has sold several million breast self-examination teaching models. The small lifelike model included with this book can literally save lives.

At WRS Publishing, we are only interested in producing books that we can be proud of—books that focus on people and/or issues that enlighten and inspire, books that change lives for the better. **Call us toll-free at 1-800-299-3366 for suggestions or for a free book catalog.**

WATCH FOR THESE OTHER WRS TITLES:

WOULD YOU GIVE TWO MINUTES A DAY FOR A LIFETIME OF LOVE? A life plan designed to help couples develop a clear focus for their lives together. With the right information and skills, couples will develop a vision of shared hopes, dreams and goals.

SALESPEAK: EVERYBODY SELLS SOMETHING How to boost your career and your income by effectively selling yourself and your ideas, from one of America's top young women speakers. A must-read for anyone who speaks in front of an audience—from the corporate executive to the PTA volunteer.

THE HEALING ARTS – From 70 living American artists, this book represents the best from a renowned collection of art dedicated to the heritage of medicine.

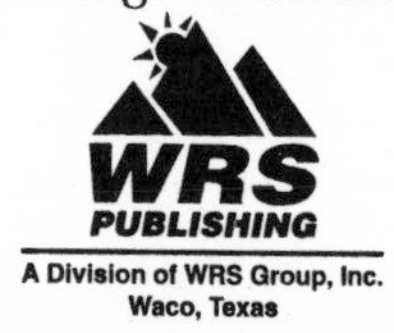

A Division of WRS Group, Inc.
Waco, Texas